Getting Ready for My Dental Surgery

Dental Procedure Under Anesthesia for Kids – Preparation and Recovery

This book belongs to:

Written by Dr. Fei Zheng-Ward   Illustrated by Moch. Fajar Shobaru

Copyright © 2025 Fei Zheng-Ward

All rights reserved. Published by Fei Zheng-Ward, an imprint of FZWbooks. No part of this book may be copied, reproduced, recorded, transmitted, or stored by any means or in any form, electronic or mechanical, without obtaining prior written permission from the copyright owner.

Identifiers: ISBN 979-8-89318-117-3 (eBook)
　　　　　　　　ISBN 979-8-89318-118-0 (paperback)
　　　　　　　　ISBN 979-8-89318-119-7 (hardcover)

Your dentist or oral surgeon is a special doctor who helps take care of your teeth, gums, and mouth.

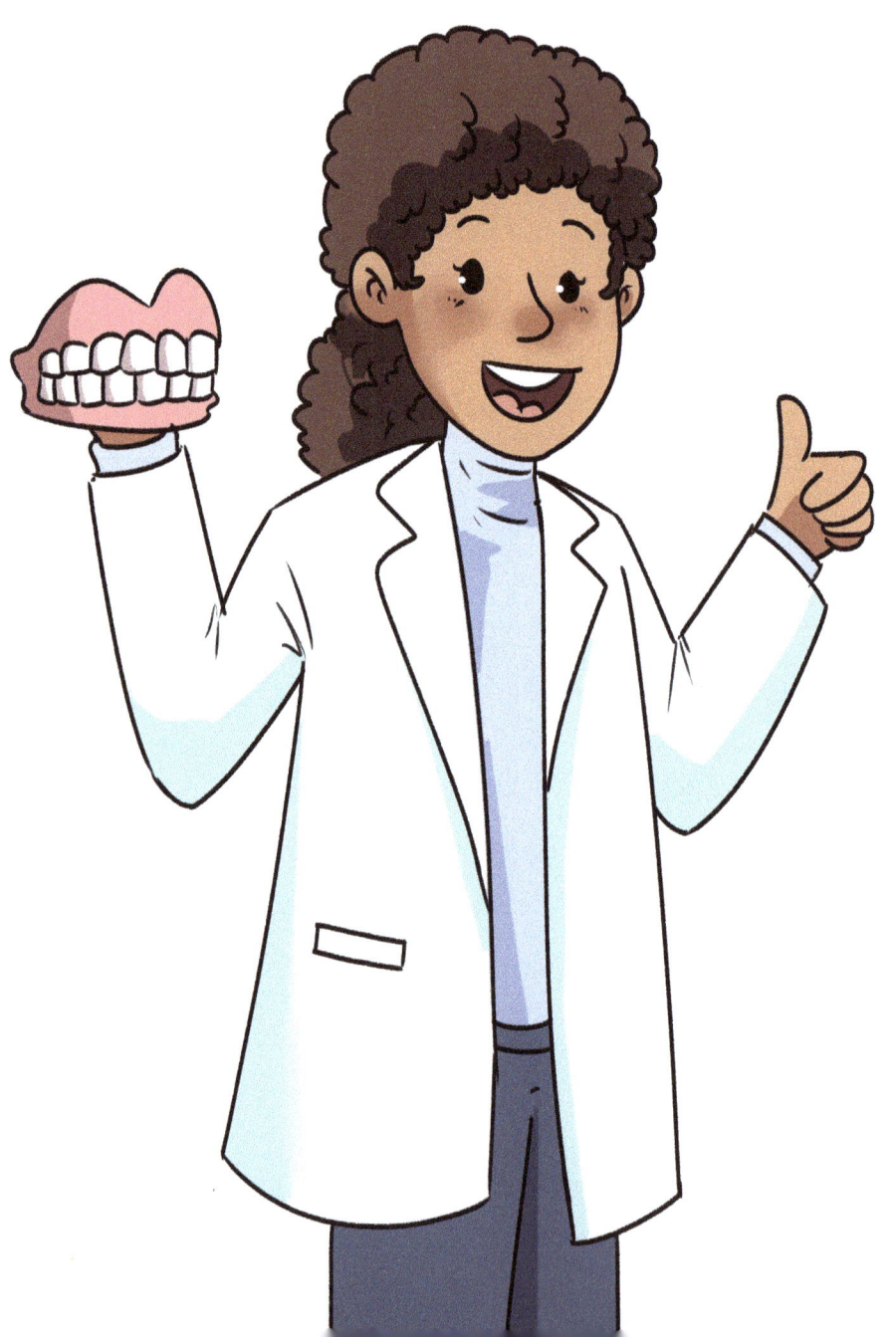

They help keep everything healthy and strong so you can eat your favorite foods, say your favorite words, and show off your big, beautiful smile!

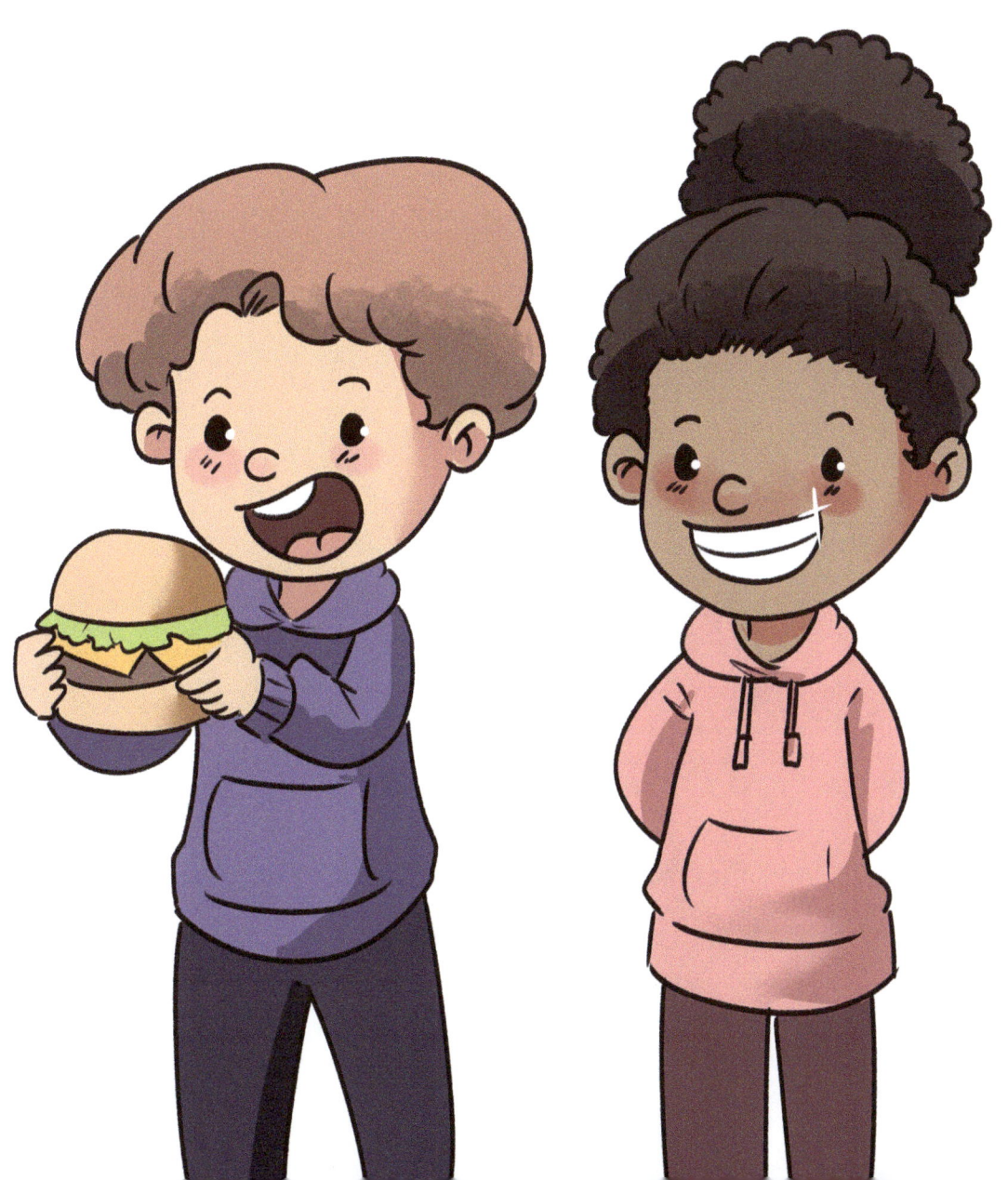

On the day of your dental surgery,
you will need to skip breakfast.
That's how your body knows it's time to get ready!

You can bring something special from home like
your favorite toy or blanket.

It's okay to feel a little nervous.

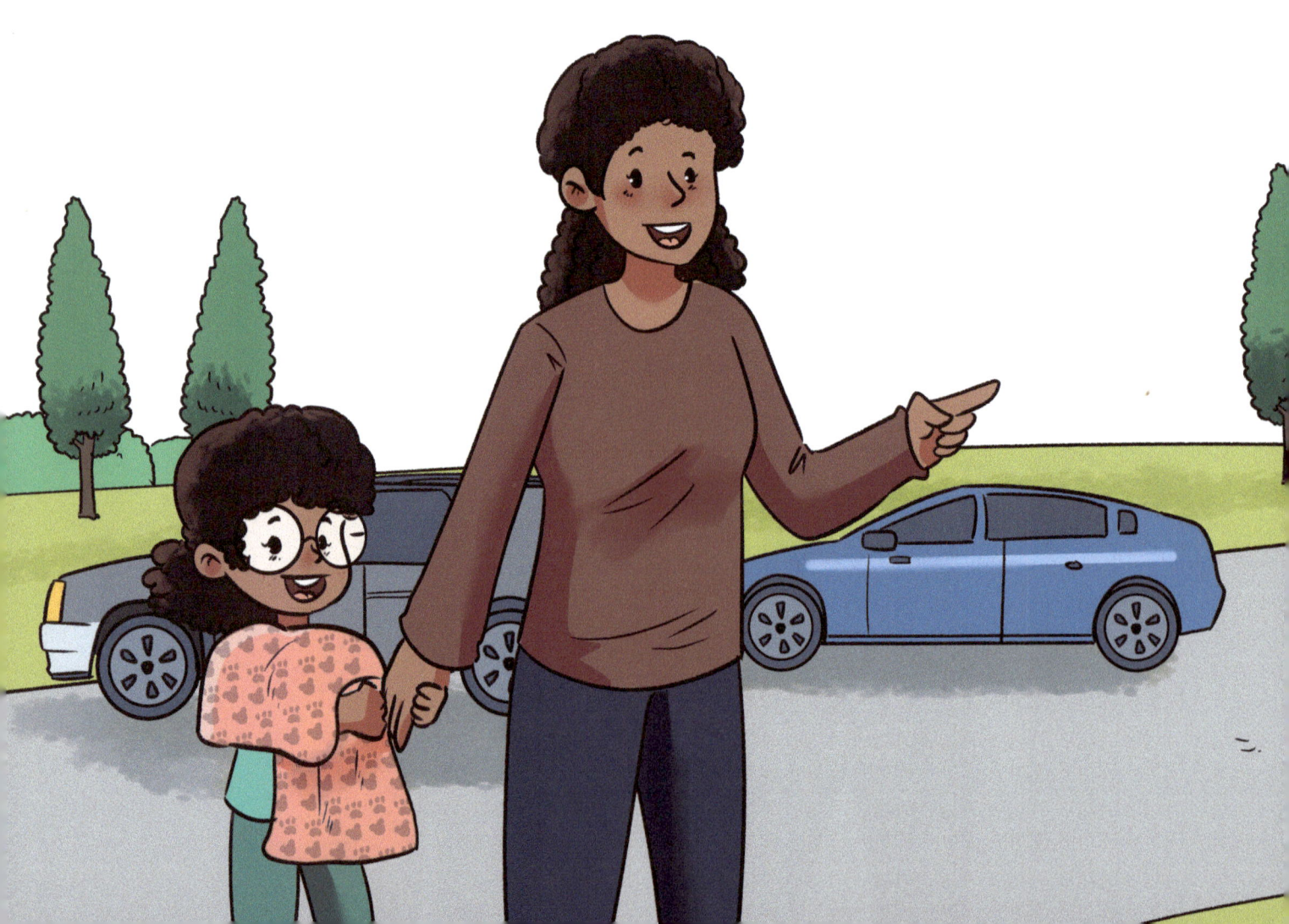

What would you like to bring with you?

Circle your answer below.

Blanket   **Toy**   **Book**   **Other:**_____

You'll check in and tell them your name and birthday.

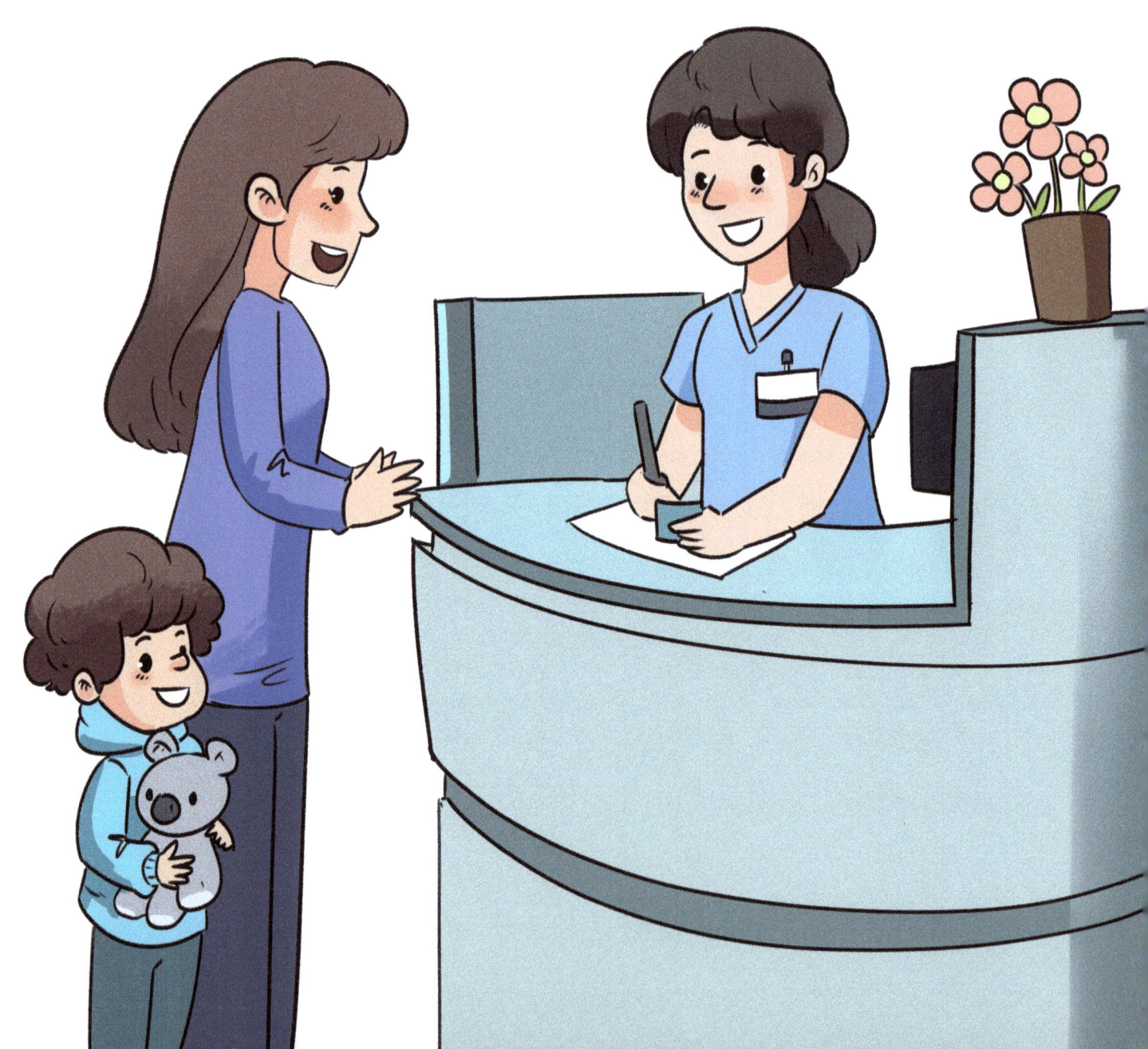

Then, you will receive a special wristband.
Now everyone will know your name.

What color wristband will you get?
Circle the color of your wristband below.

Red   Green   Yellow

Blue   Pink   Orange

Purple   Black   White

Other: _____

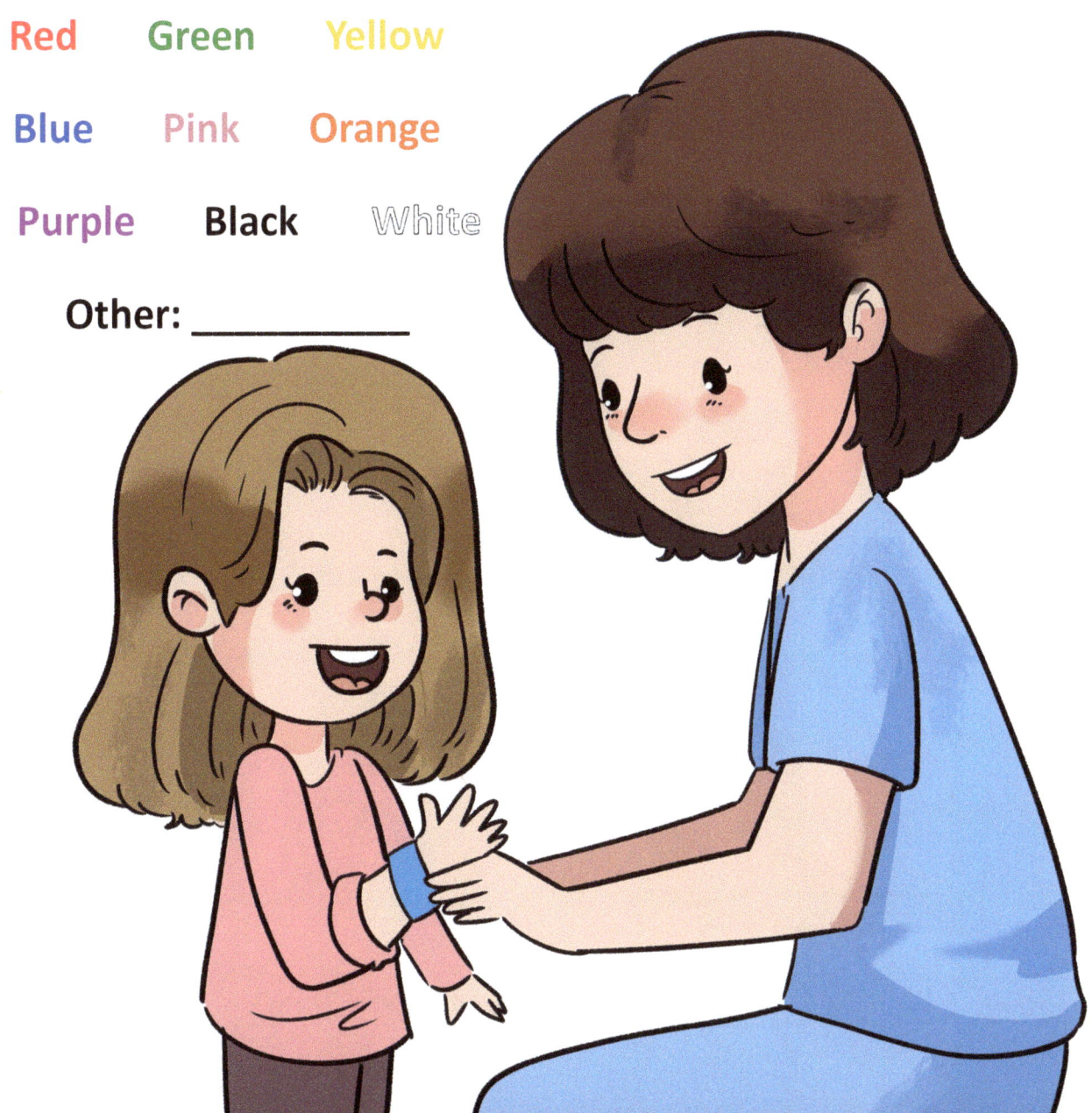

They will check your weight and height before getting you ready.

Do you know how much you weigh?

Do you know how tall you are?

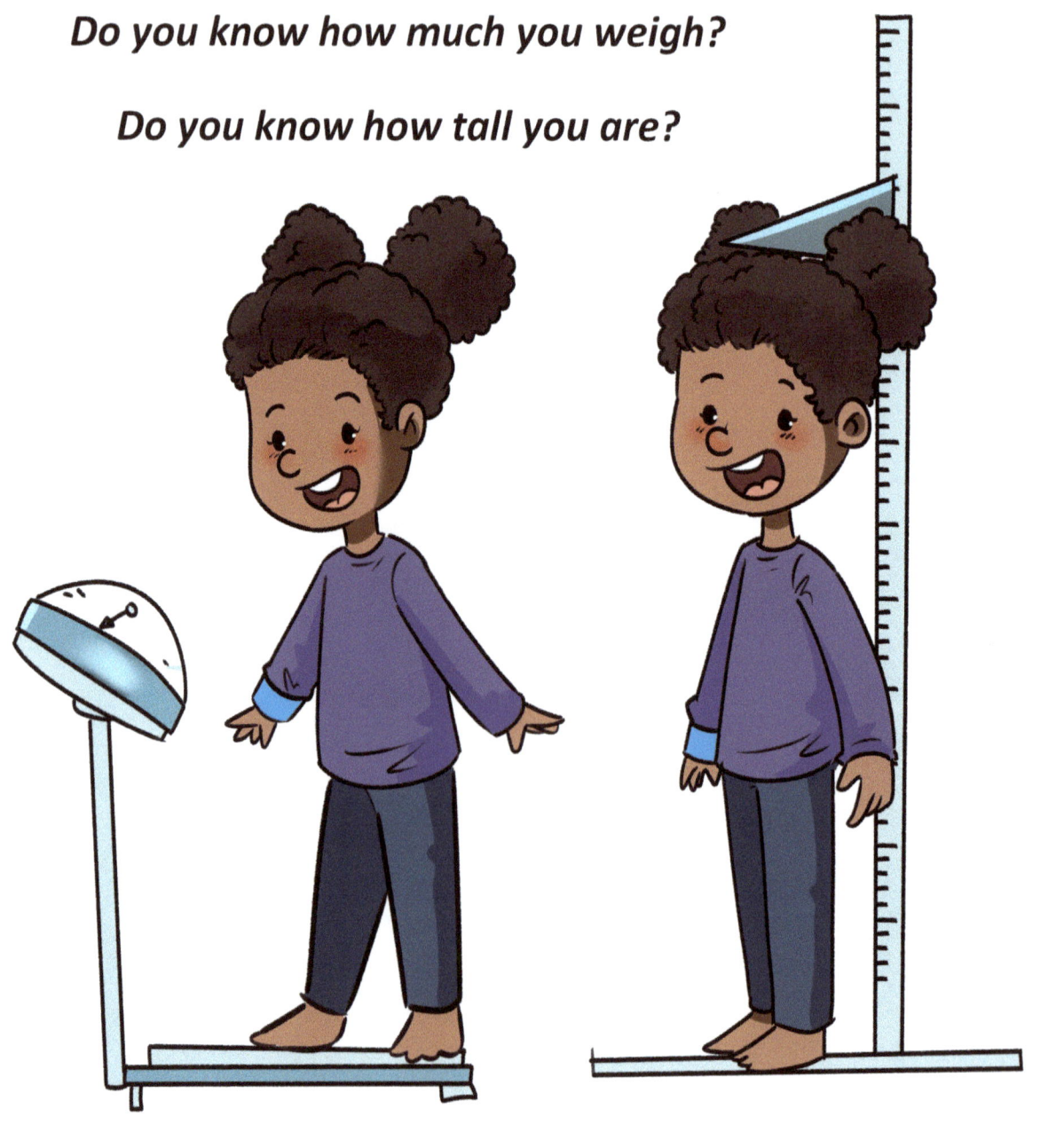

My weight is: _____   My height is: _____

You will change into a new outfit, put on a hat, a gown (that looks like a backward superhero cape), and some socks.

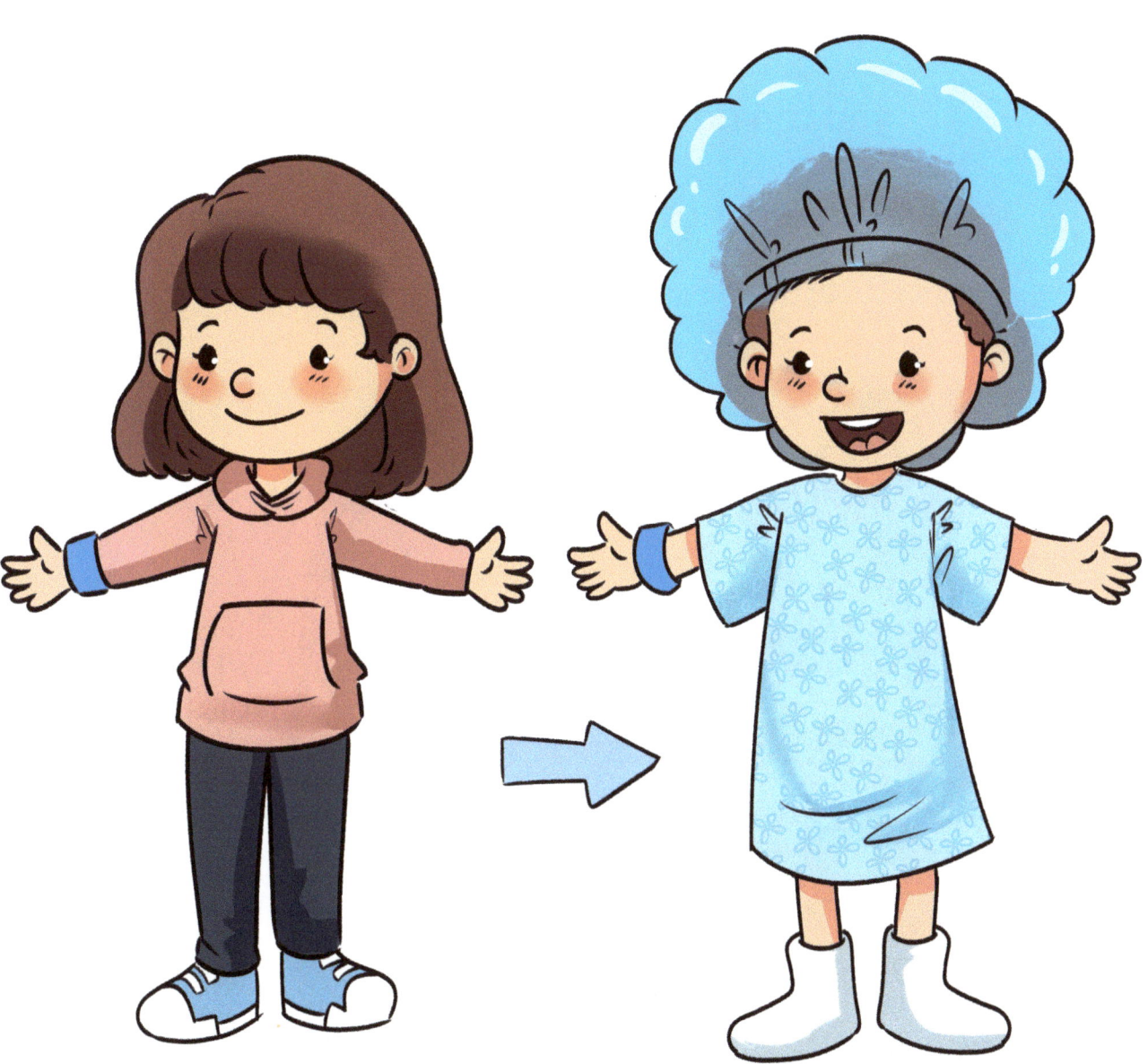

Your nurse will put a bandage-like tape or a clip on your finger or toe to see how much oxygen is in your body. Oxygen is in the air you breathe. It helps your body work so you can do all the things you love!

Which finger or toe do you want to use?

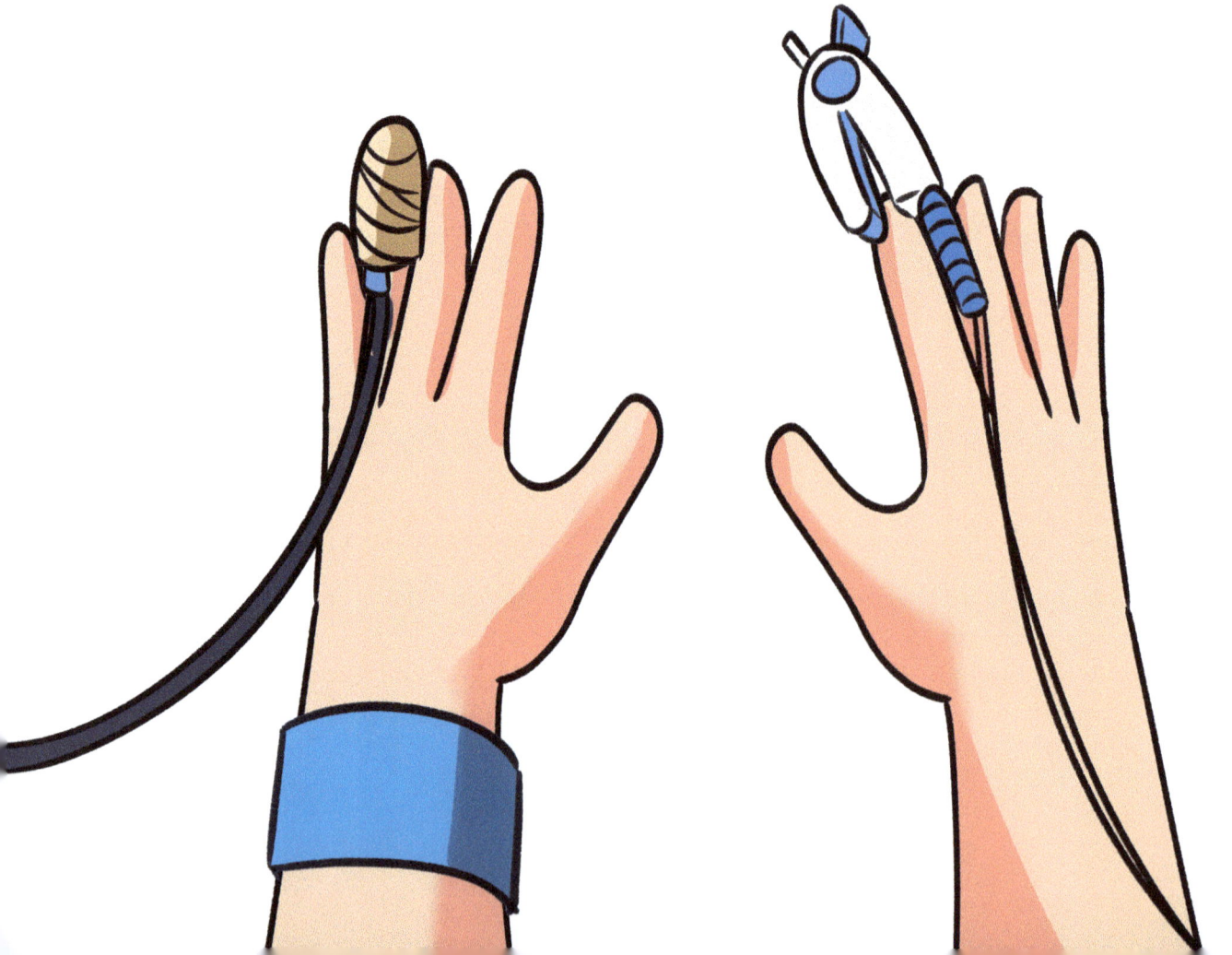

You'll get a blood pressure cuff around your arm or leg.

The cuff will give you a BIG squeeze.

Don't forget to stay still while they're examining you.

Are you ready?

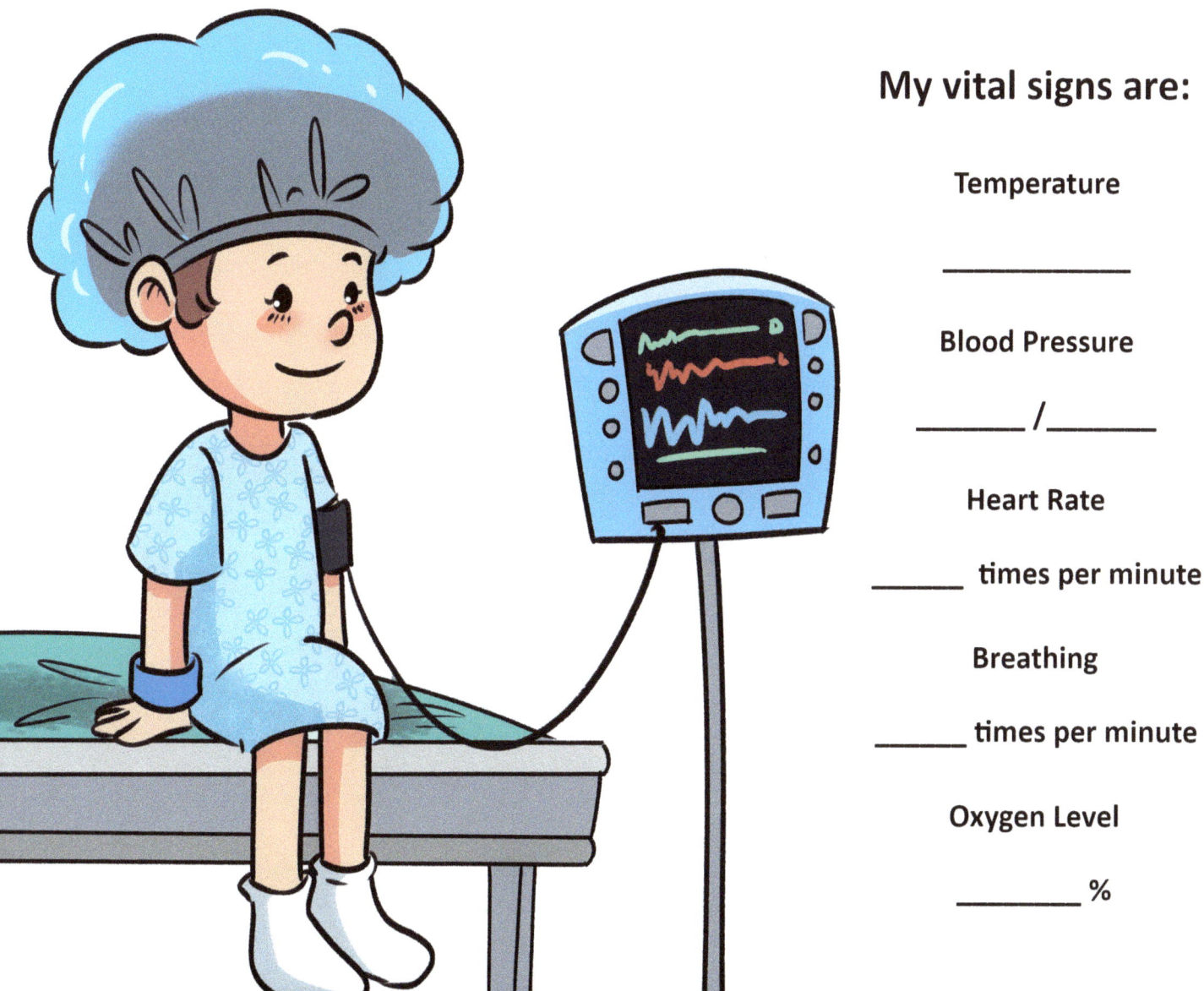

My vital signs are:

Temperature

_____

Blood Pressure

_____ / _____

Heart Rate

_____ times per minute

Breathing

_____ times per minute

Oxygen Level

_____ %

You and your parent or guardian will meet your dentist
(or oral surgeon) and anesthesia doctor.
They're gentle, kind, and here to help you feel better.

Your doctors are happy to answer any questions you have.

If you have any questions, feel free to ask!

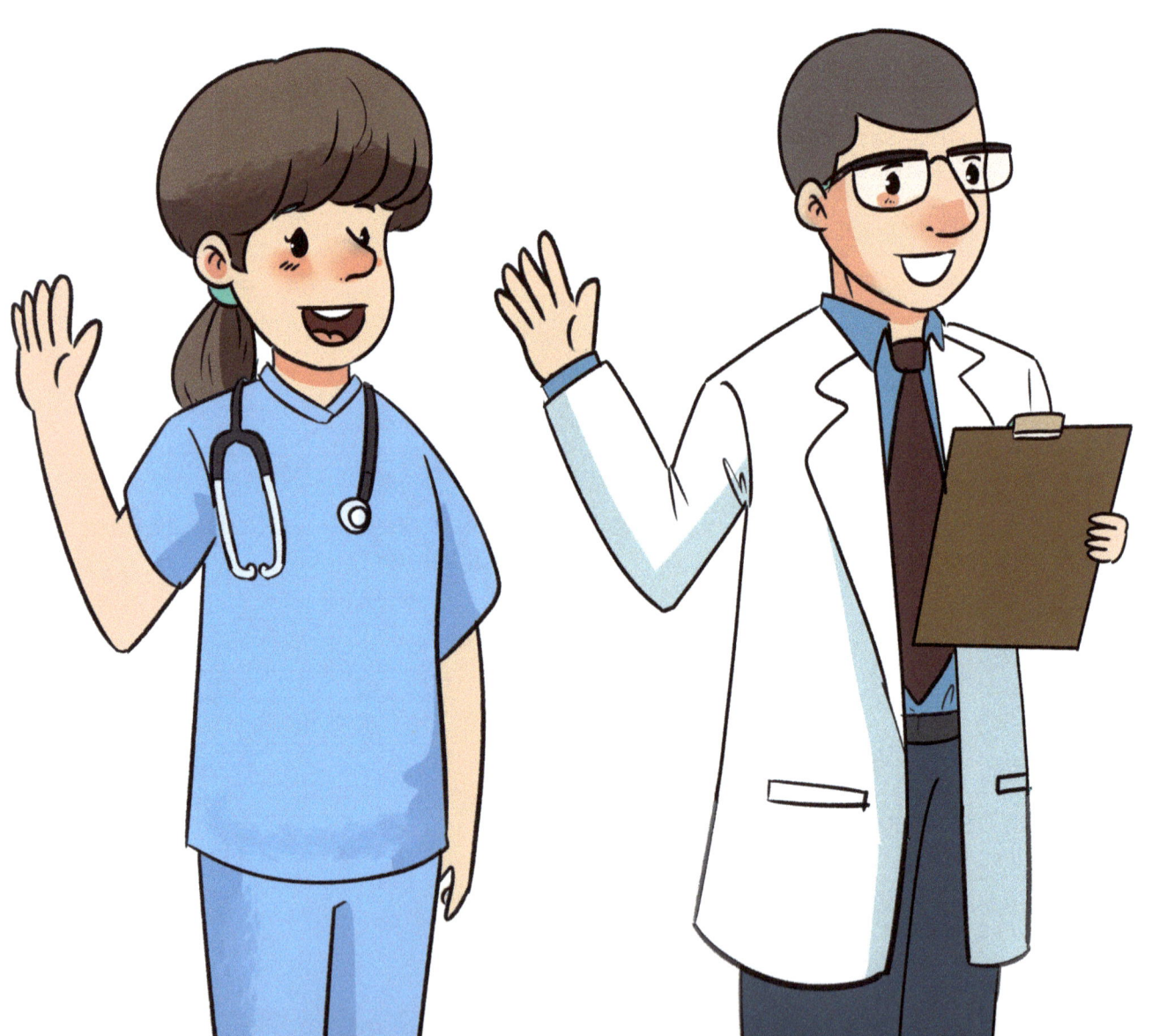

Everyone is here to help you feel comfortable and safe.

If you feel a little nervous, your doctor might give you some special medicine to help you feel calm and relaxed.

You've got this!

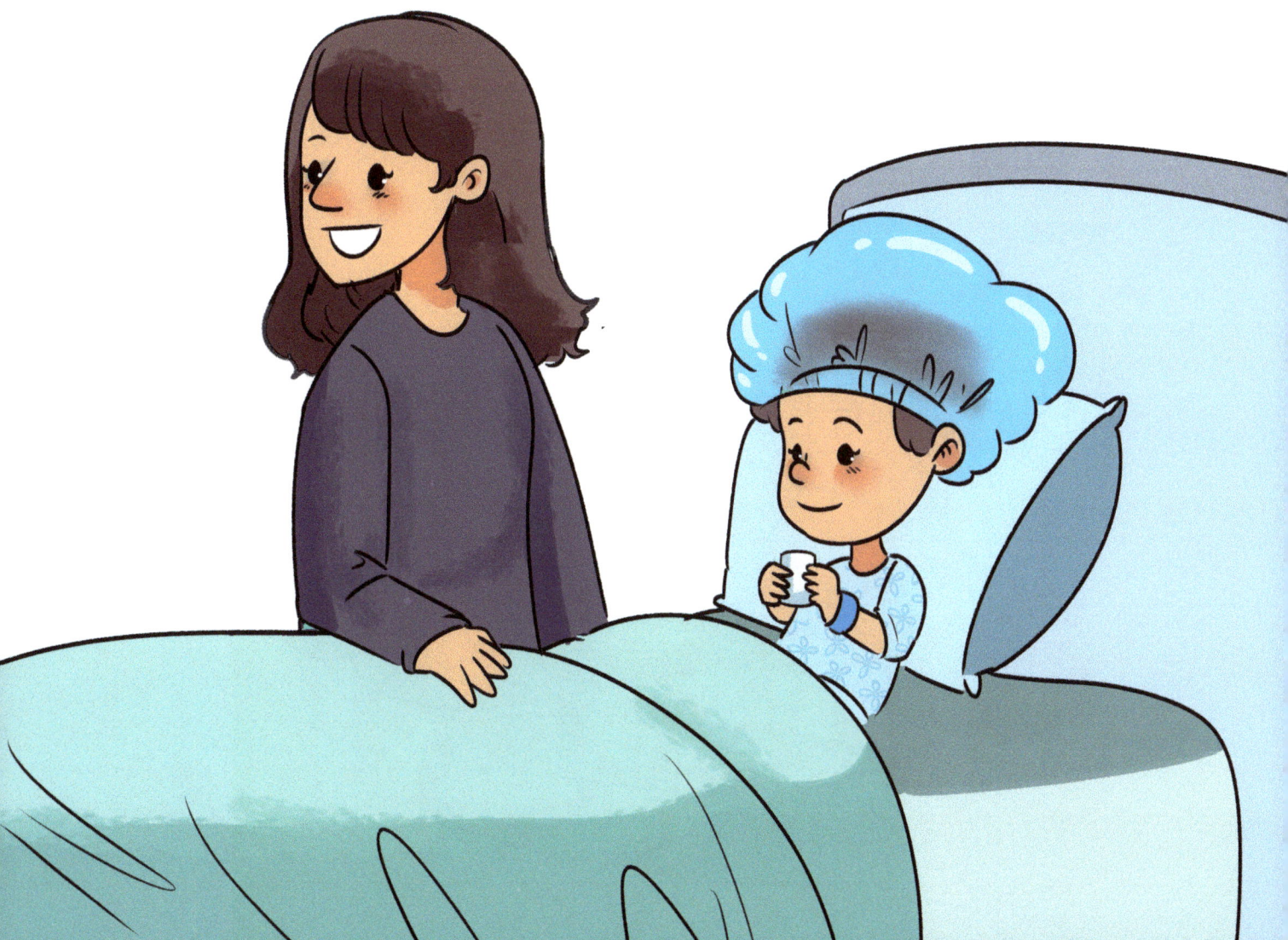

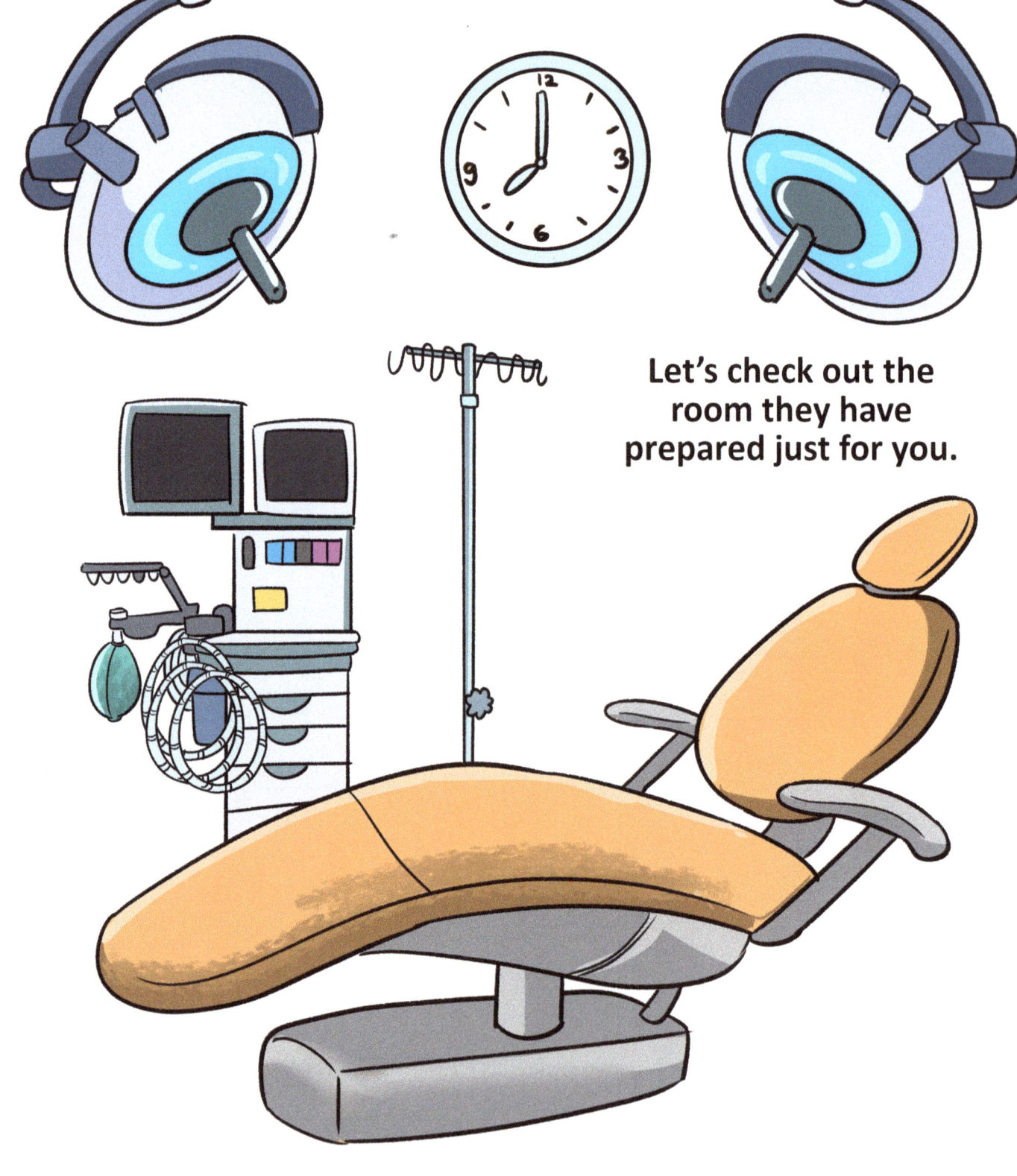
Let's check out the room they have prepared just for you.

Can you find these things in the room?

1. A comfy chair in the middle of the room just for you
2. Friendly staff wearing masks who will help with your surgery
3. Bright lights hanging from the ceiling
4. An IV (intravenous) pole for hanging bags of fluids and medicine
5. An anesthesia machine with an attached balloon
6. A computer monitor
7. A clock on the wall

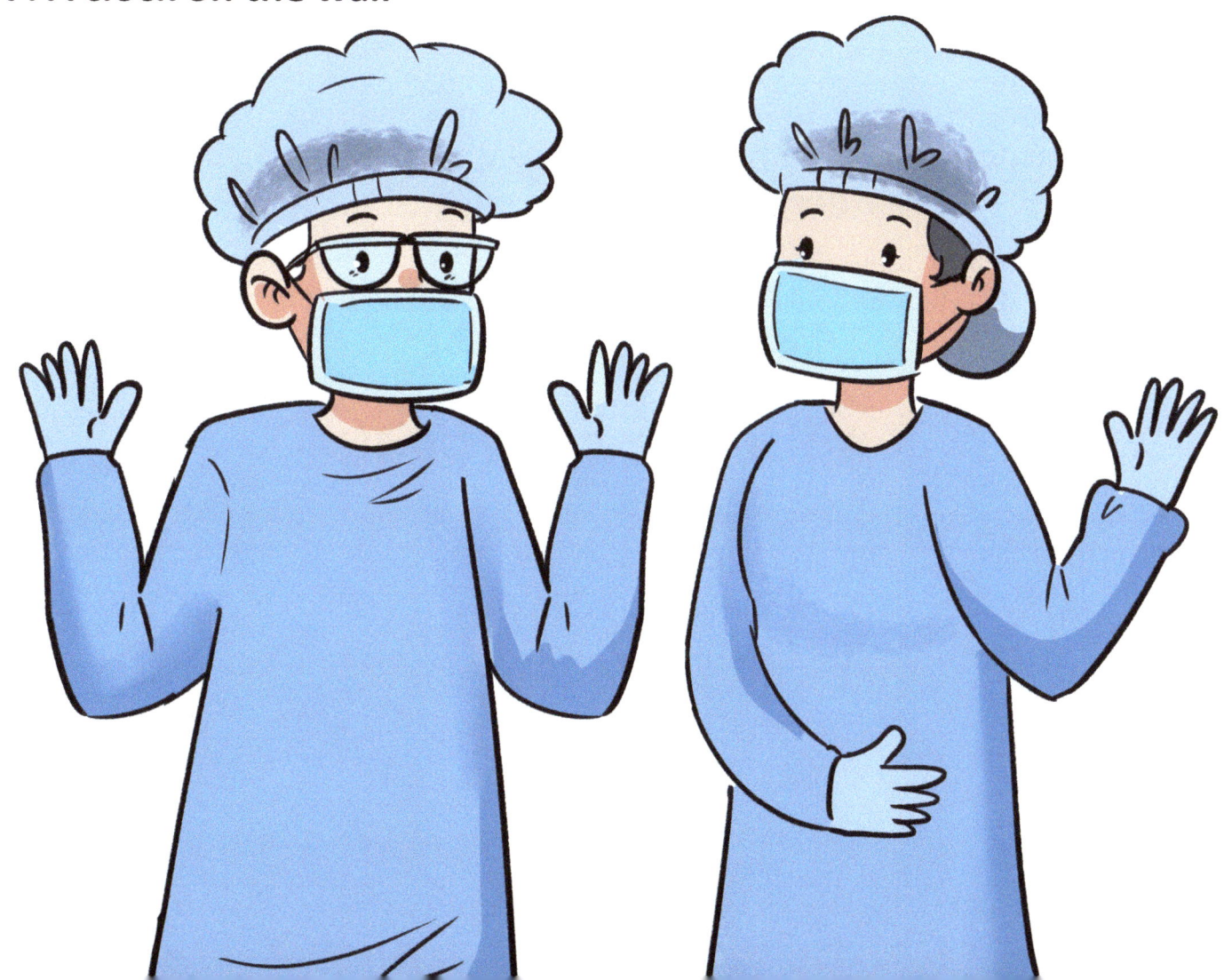

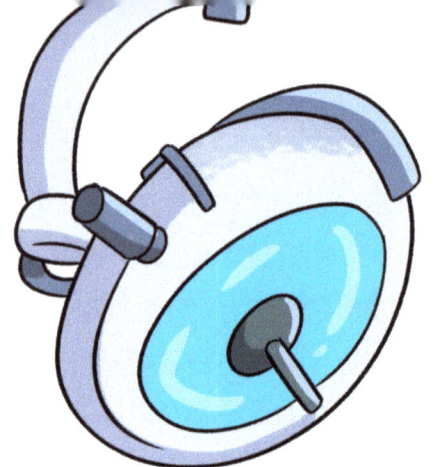

After you get on the chair, they will check your heart, breathing, blood pressure, and oxygen.

Small stickers called electrodes will be placed on your body to check your heart.

You are so brave!

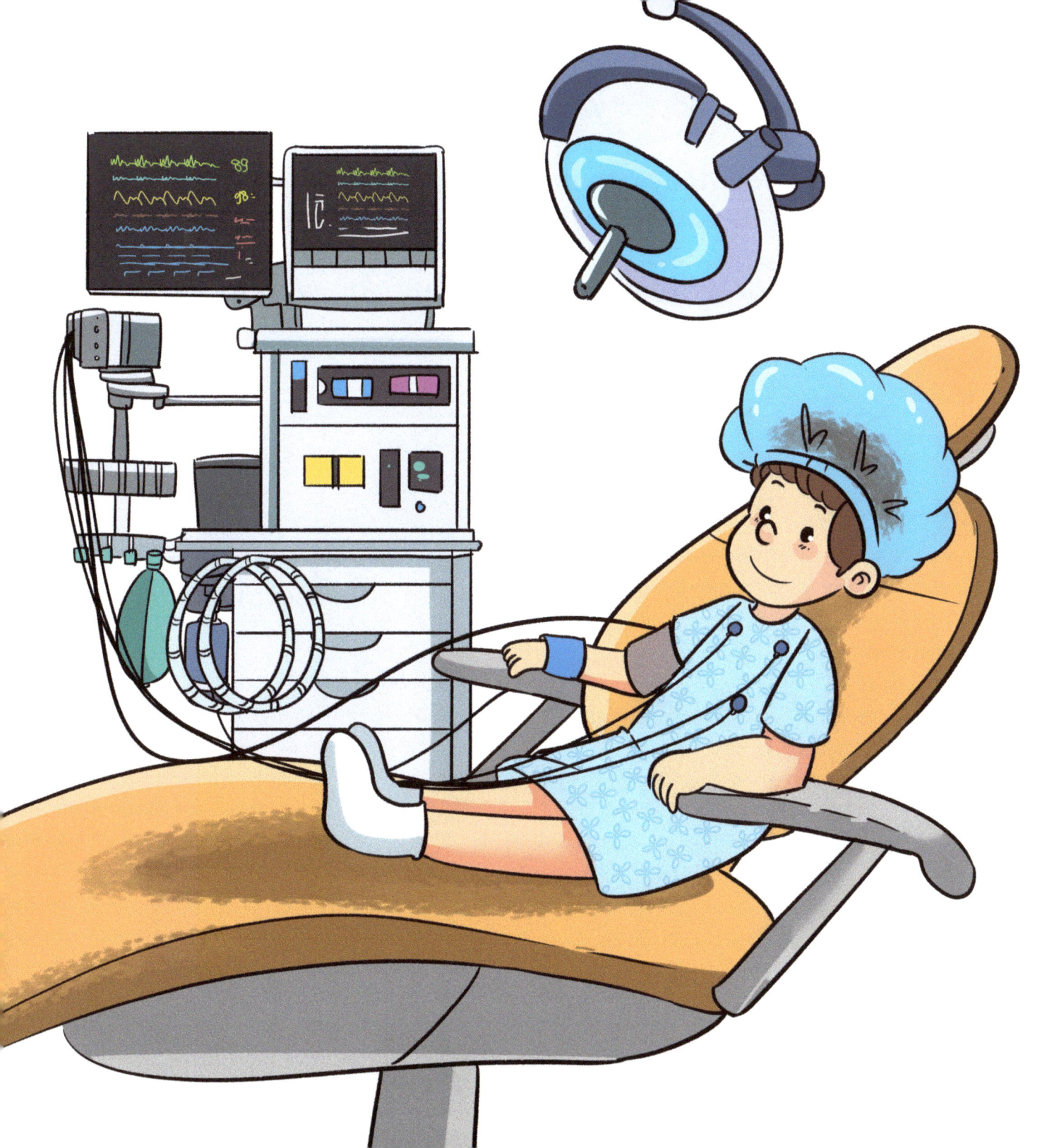

Your anesthesia doctor will give you a mask to breathe into.

Did you know they can make your mask smell sweet and delicious like bubble gum or your favorite fruit?

Draw or write down what scent you would like:

_____

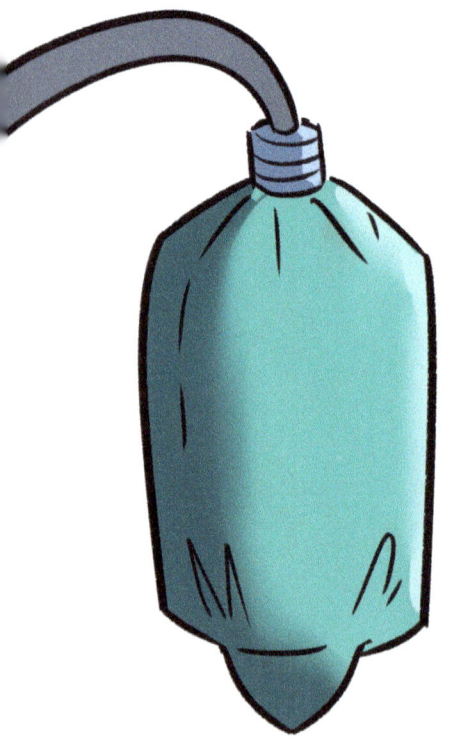

You can see your breathing by looking at the balloon attached to the anesthesia machine.

Cool, right?

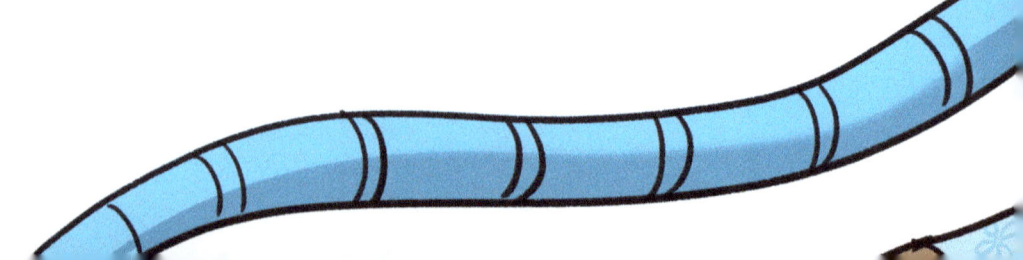

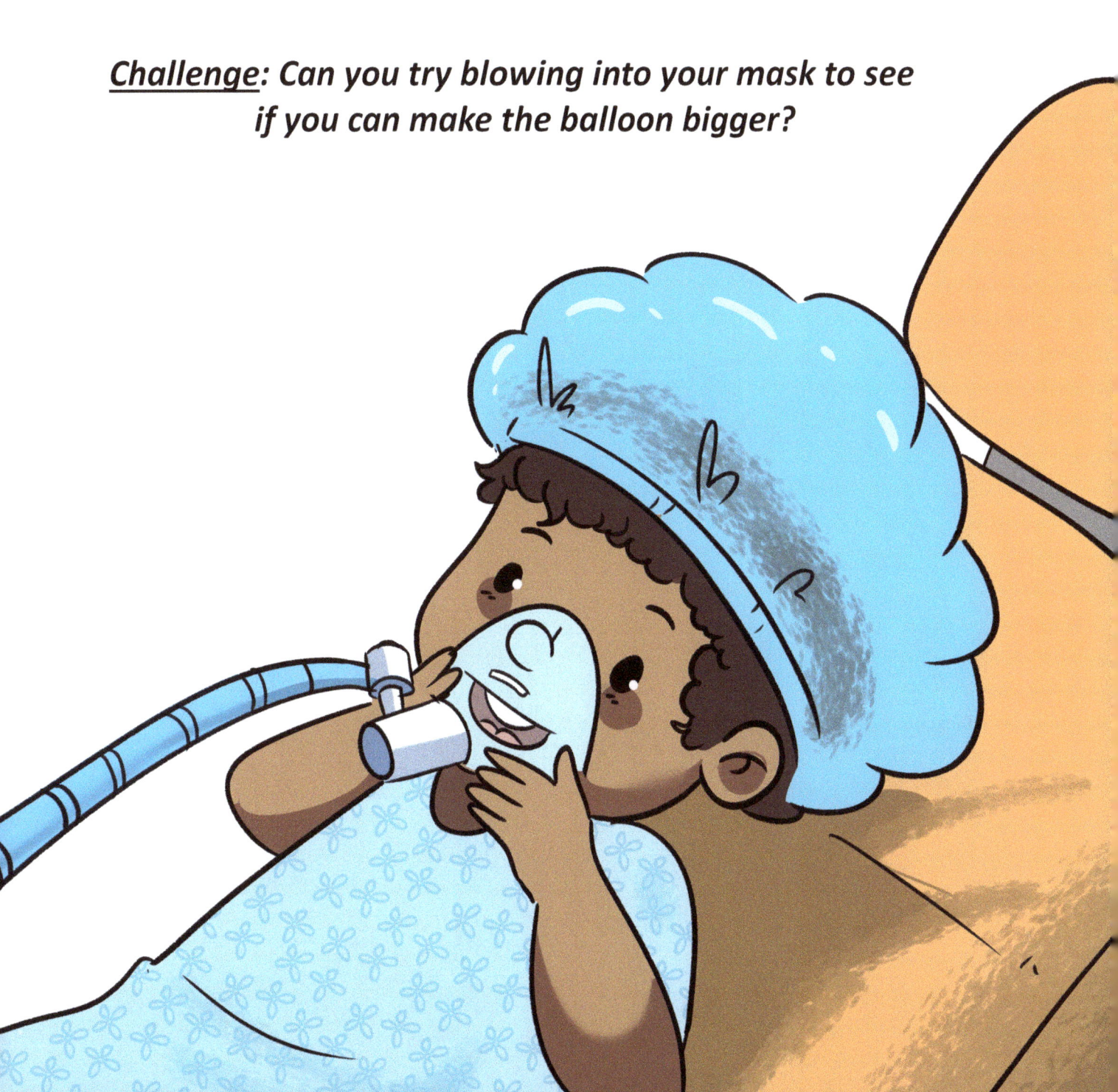

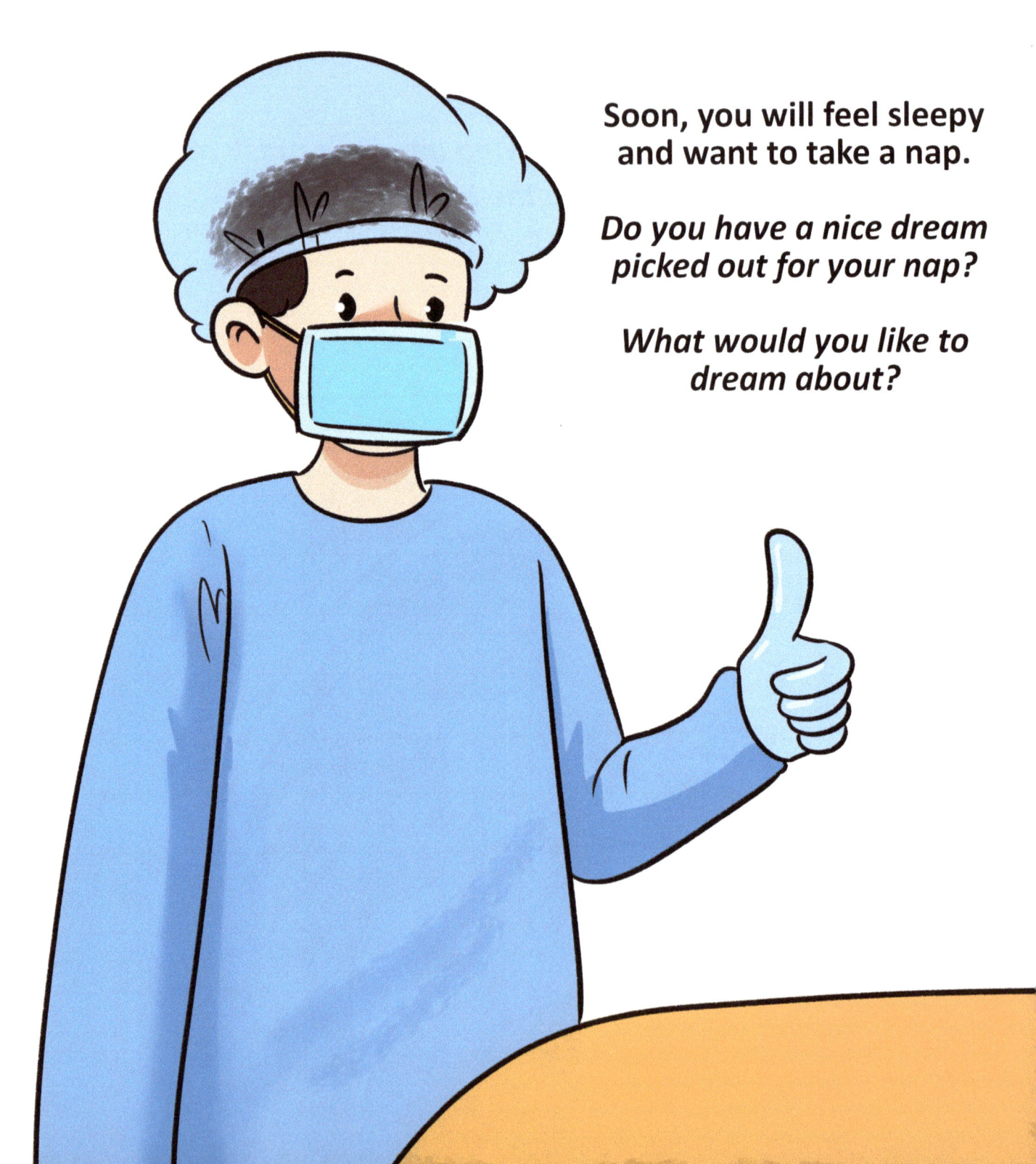

During the procedure, your dentist (or oral surgeon) will gently and carefully fix and clean your teeth, gums, or other parts of your mouth.

Your surgery will be done while you're dreaming away, and you won't feel a thing!

Your nurses and doctors will take good care of you and keep you safe and comfortable.

Sweet dreams...

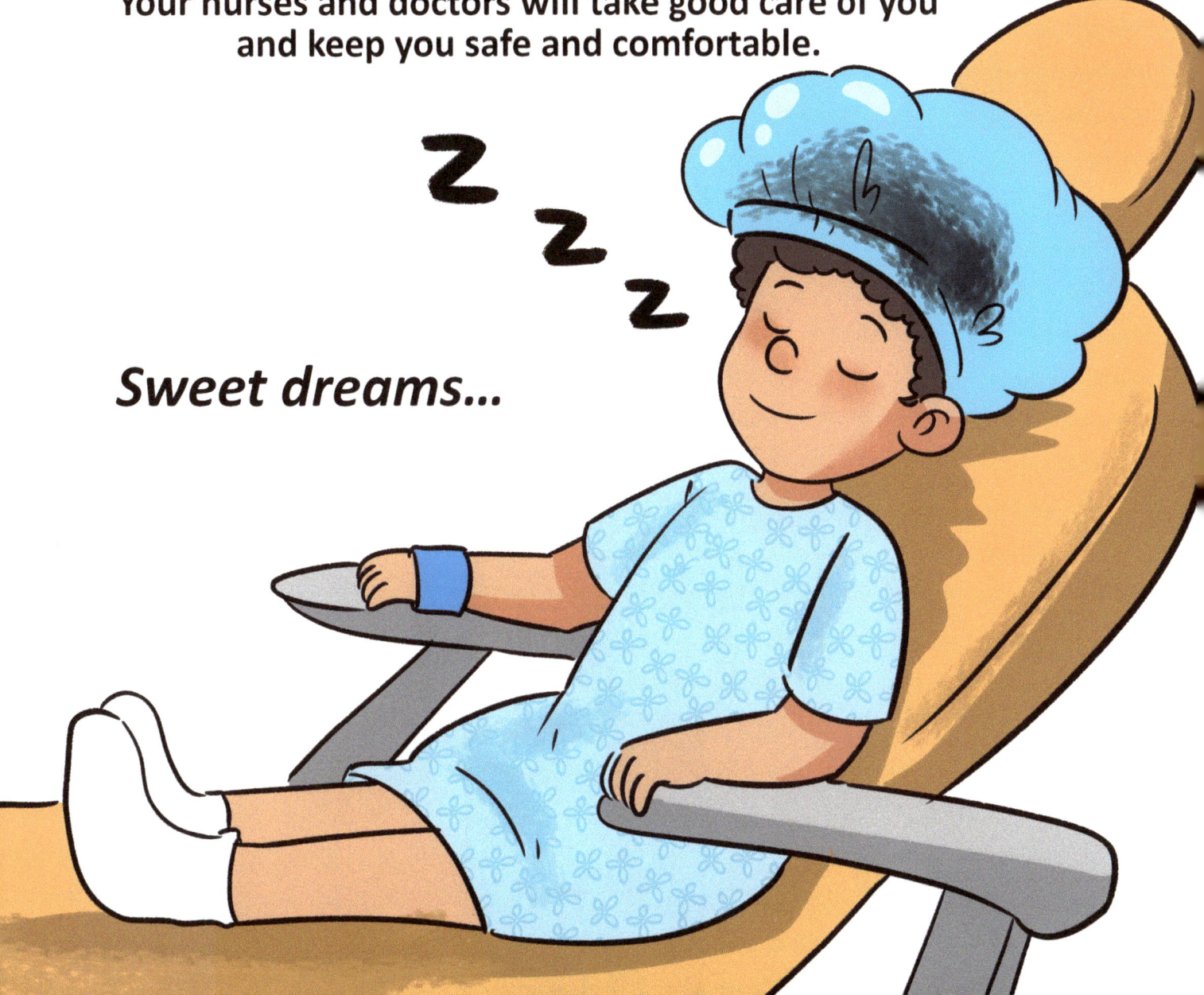

When you wake up from your nap, your surgery will be all done. Your mouth, nose, and throat may feel a little sore or uncomfortable.

If you need medicine to help you feel better, it will be given to you through the small plastic tube in your arm or leg.
The tube was placed while you were sleeping.

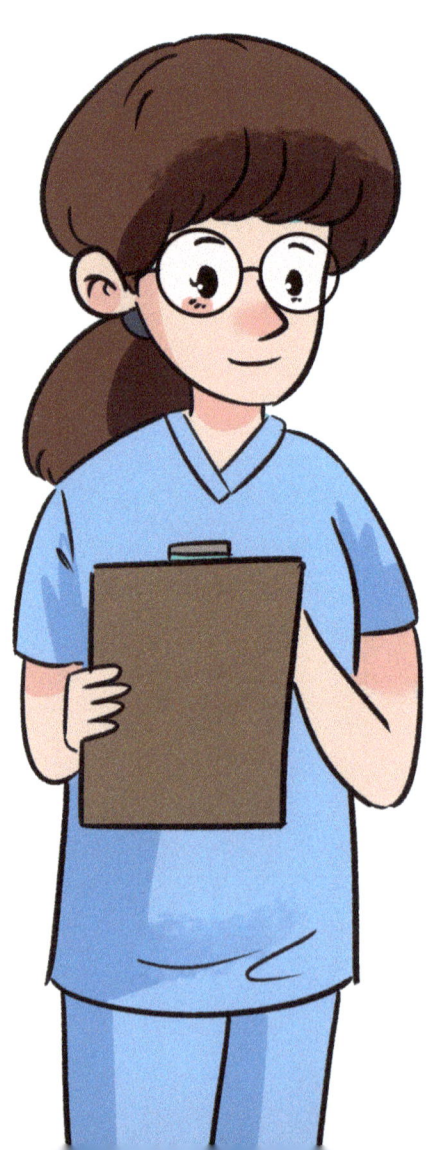

Fun fact: The small plastic tubes (also called IVs) come in different colors like yellow, blue, pink, green, gray, and orange.

What color will you get?

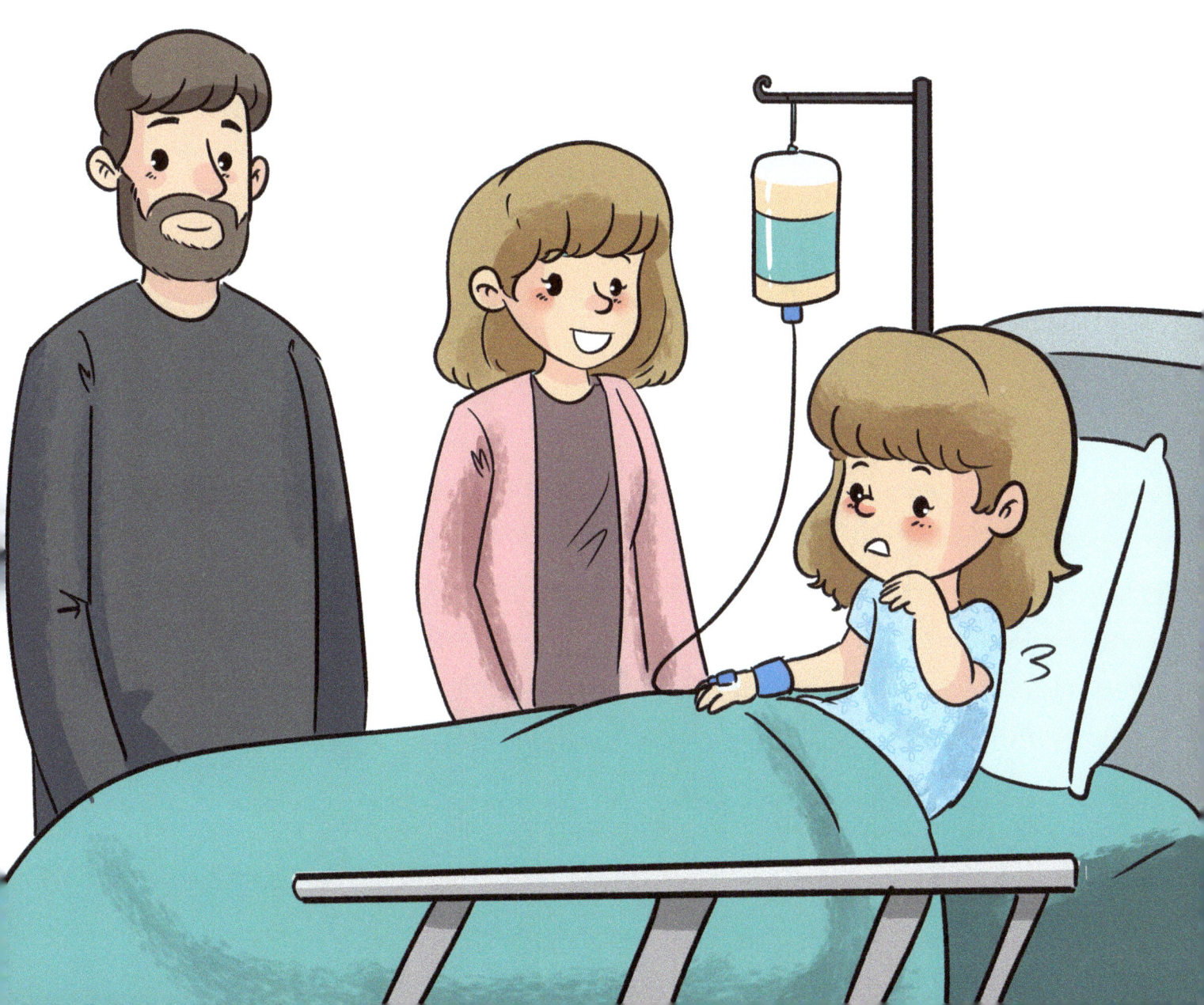

What are some things that will help you feel better and more comfortable after your dental surgery? Place a checkmark (✓) next to your favorites!

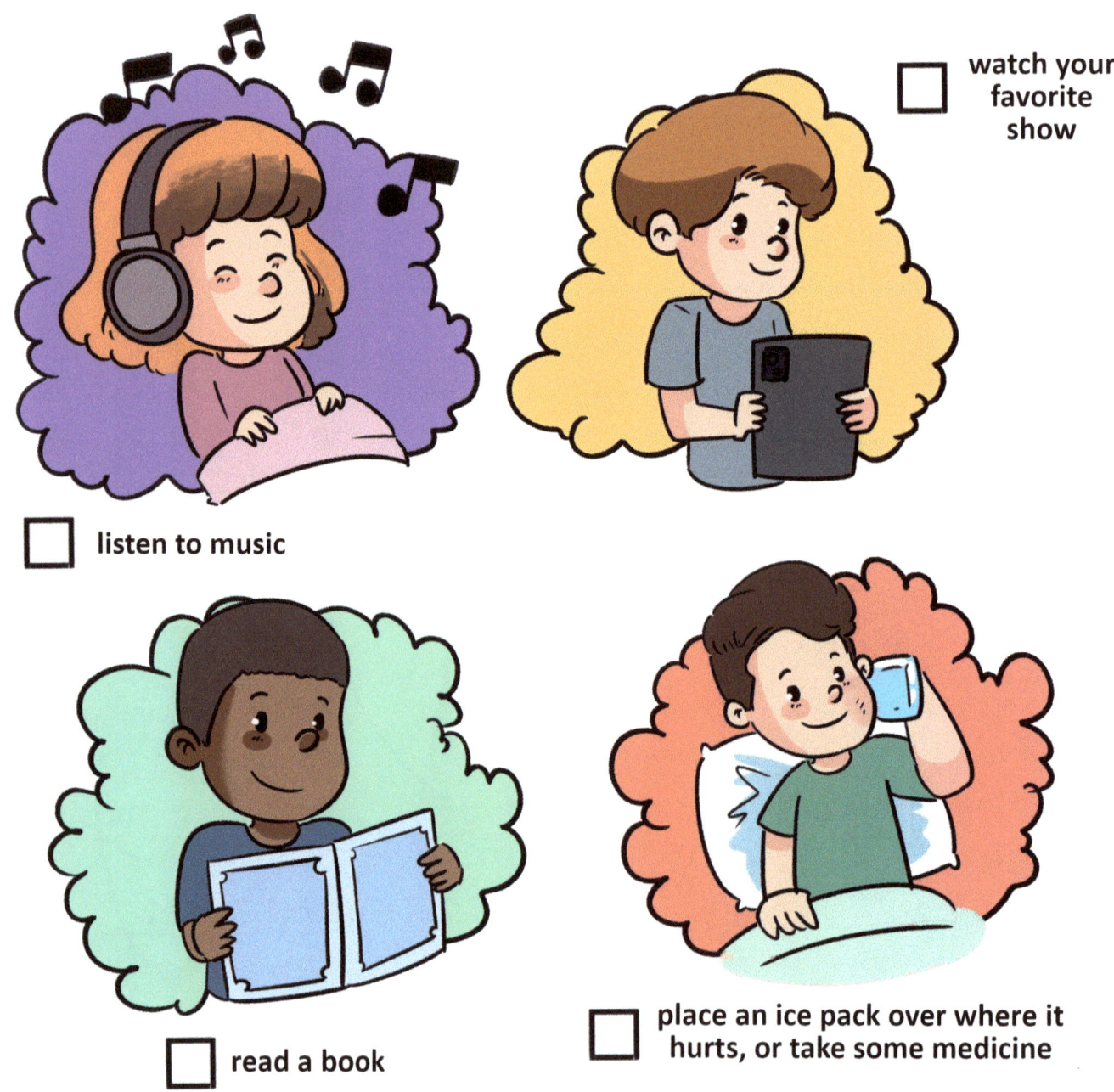

☐ watch your favorite show

☐ listen to music

☐ read a book

☐ place an ice pack over where it hurts, or take some medicine

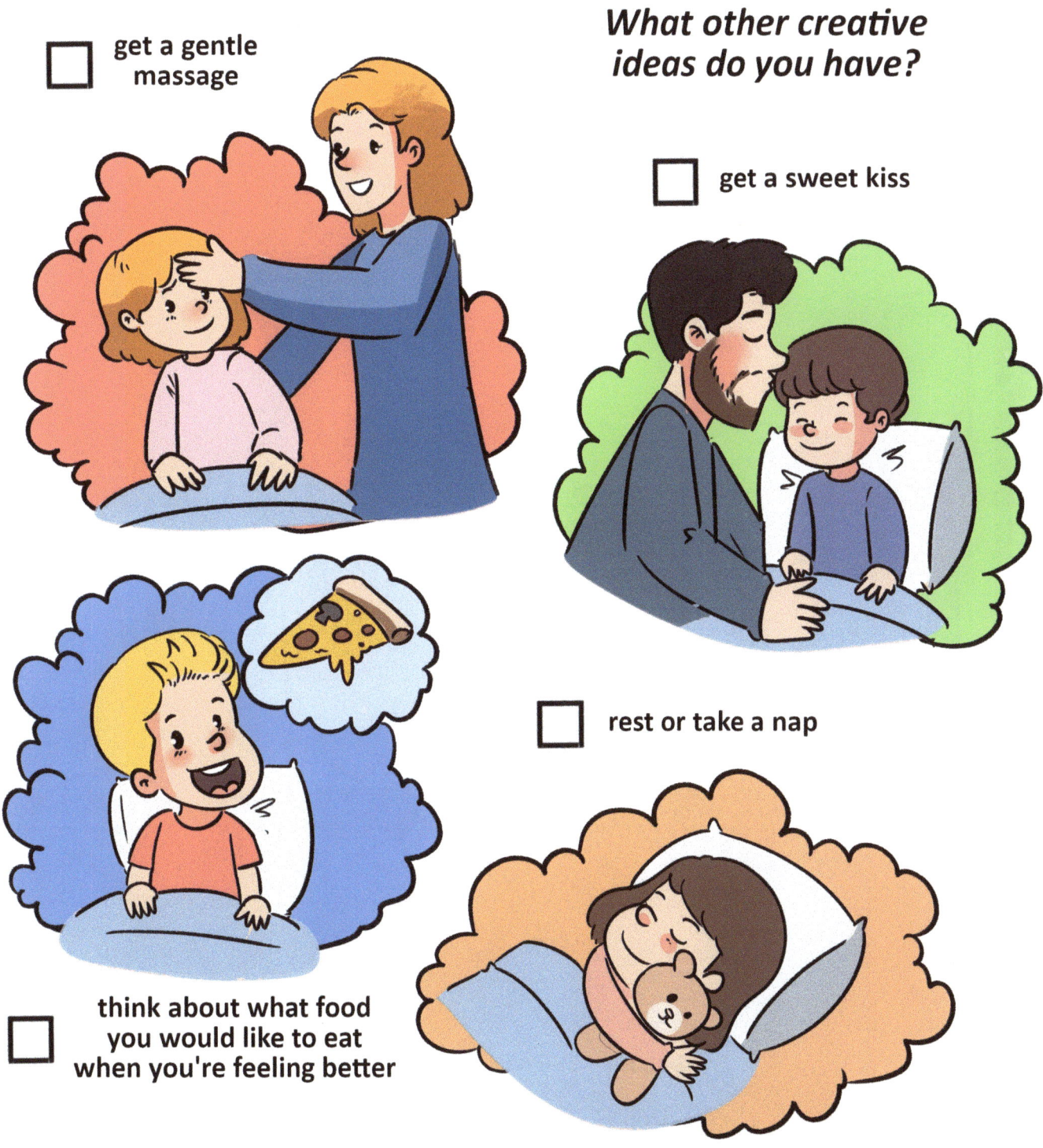

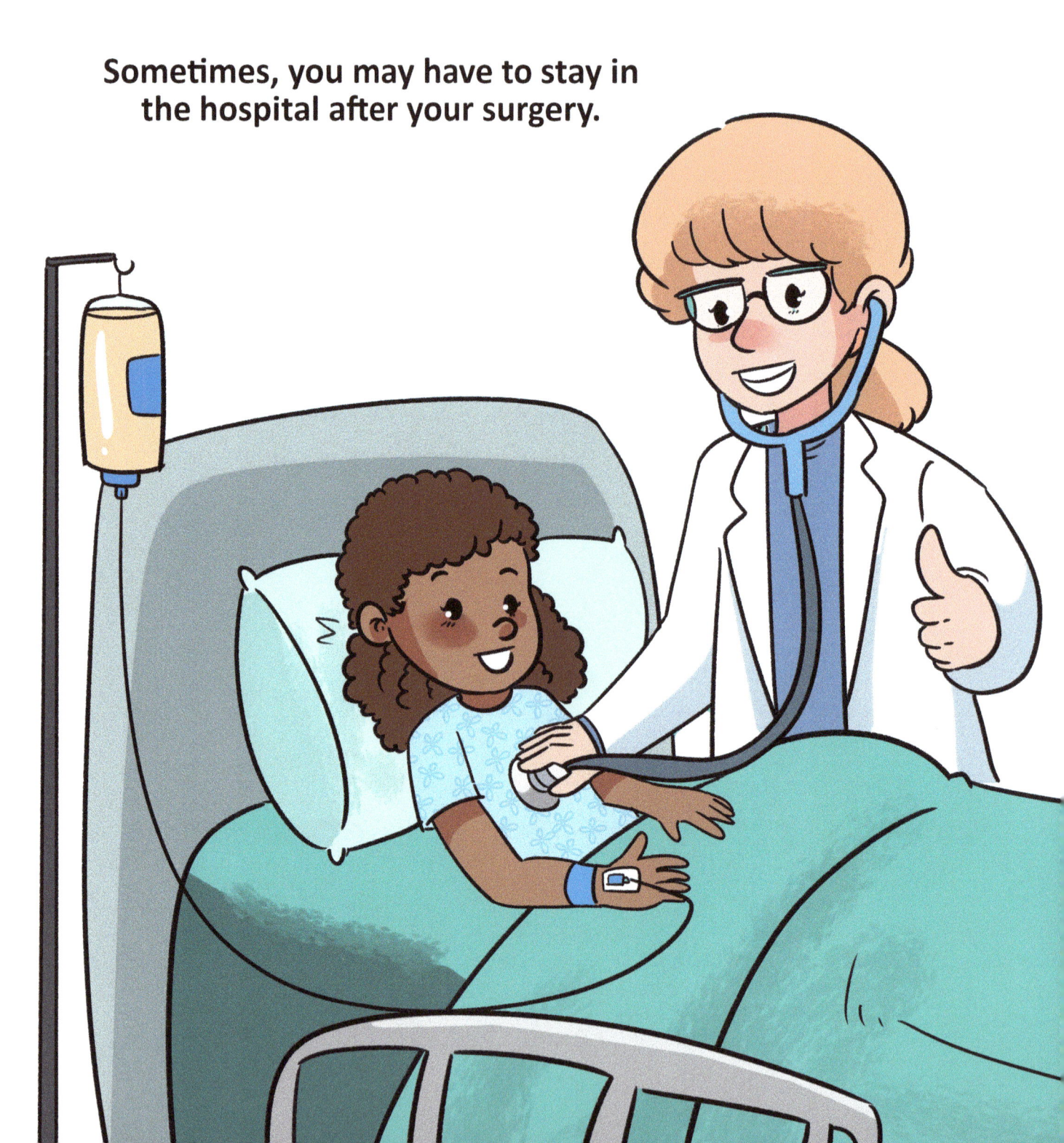

Sometimes, you may have to stay in the hospital after your surgery.

Your parent or guardian can stay with you to help you feel safe and comfortable.

When you feel better and stronger, you'll be able to continue your recovery at home.

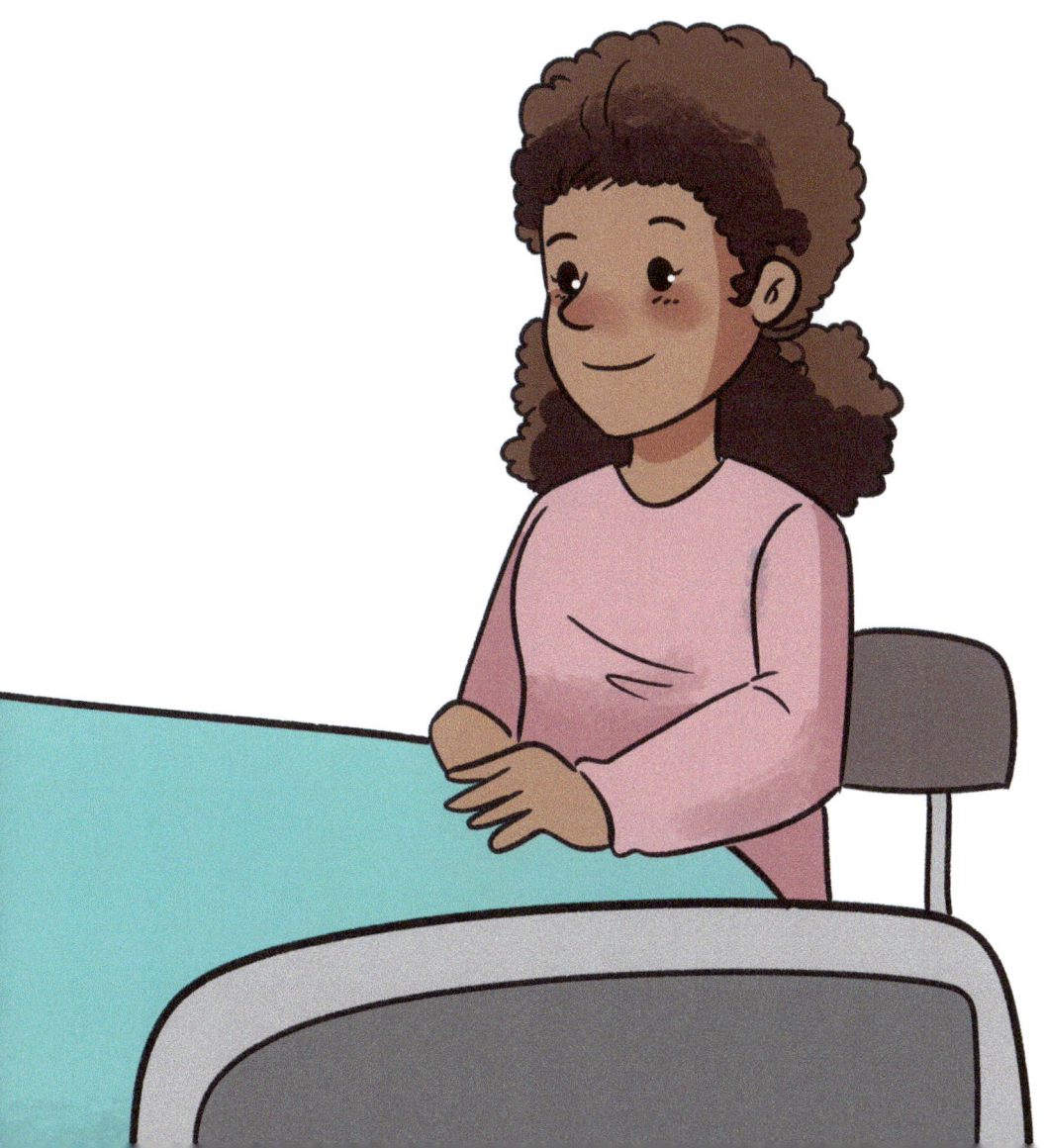

After your surgery, you might eat soft foods like smoothie, yogurt, or applesauce.

smoothie

yogurt

applesauce

What's your favorite soft food to eat?

Make a list of your favorite soft foods, and maybe go shopping with your grown-up to get ready before your surgery.

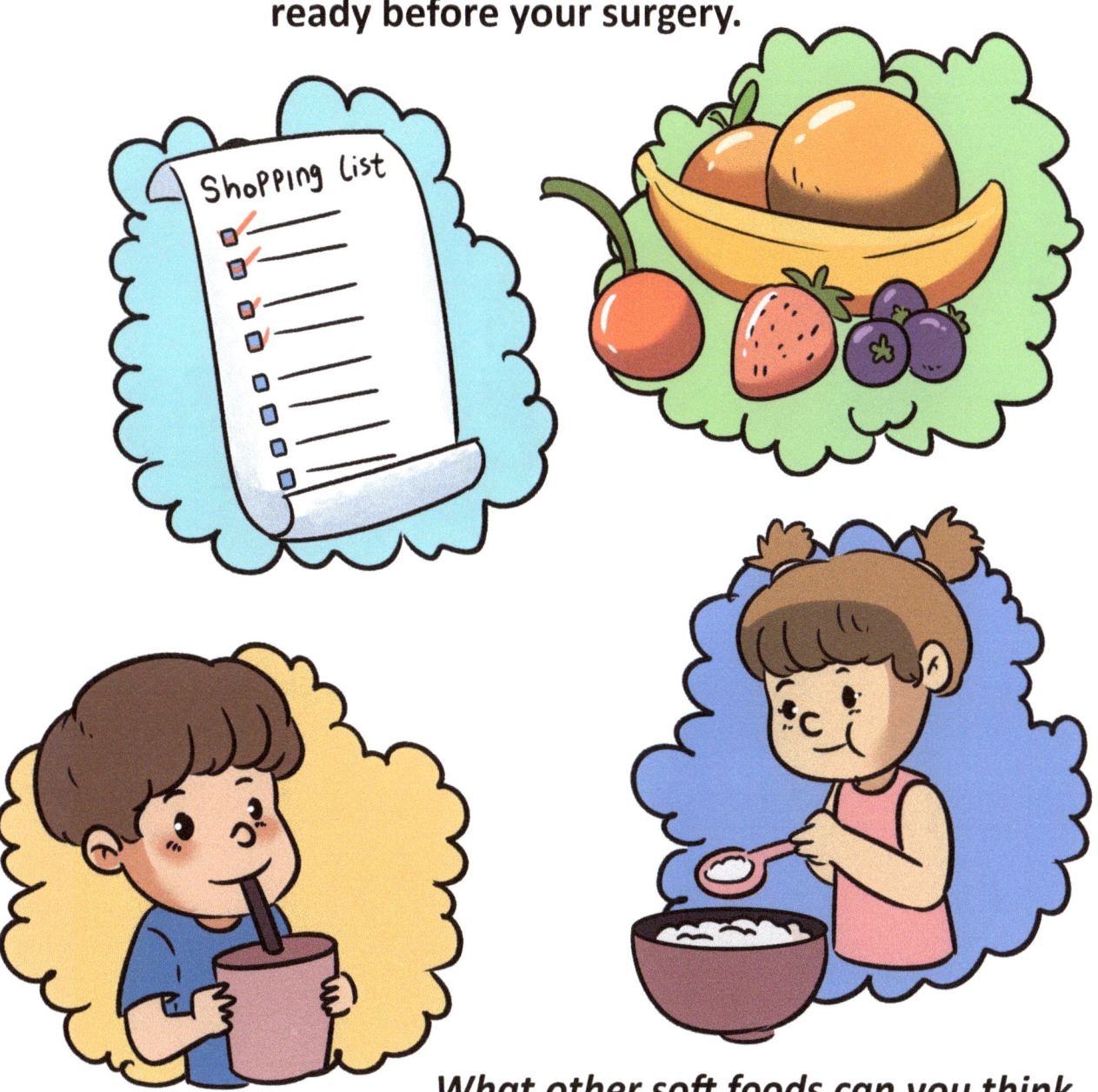

What other soft foods can you think of that you would like to eat?

While you're recovering from your surgery, please *relax* and take it easy! *What do you plan to do?*

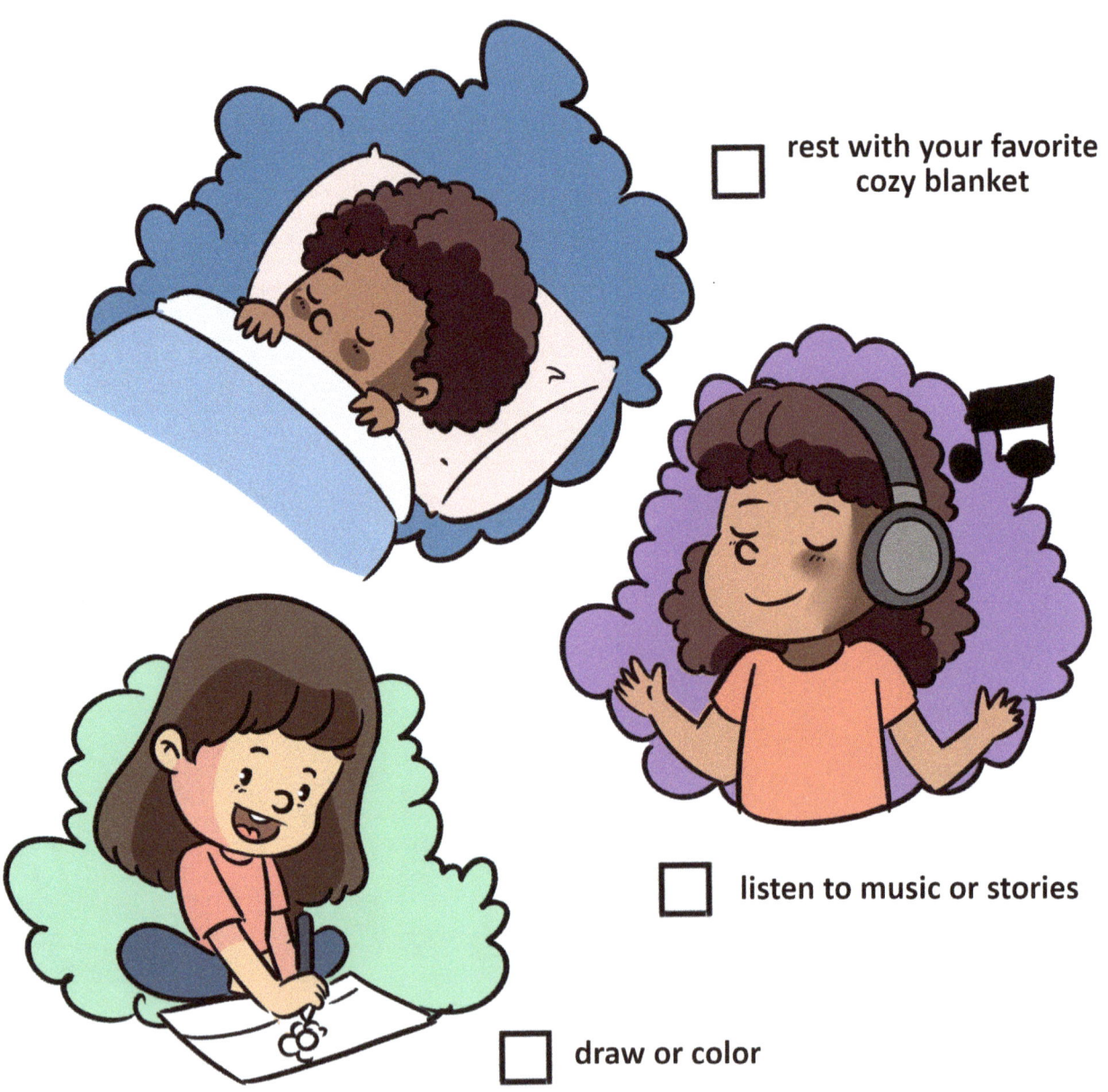

- ☐ rest with your favorite cozy blanket
- ☐ listen to music or stories
- ☐ draw or color

Take it easy, stay hydrated, and get plenty of rest to feel better and stronger.

- [ ] watch your favorite show
- [ ] read books
- [ ] play with your favorite stuffed animal

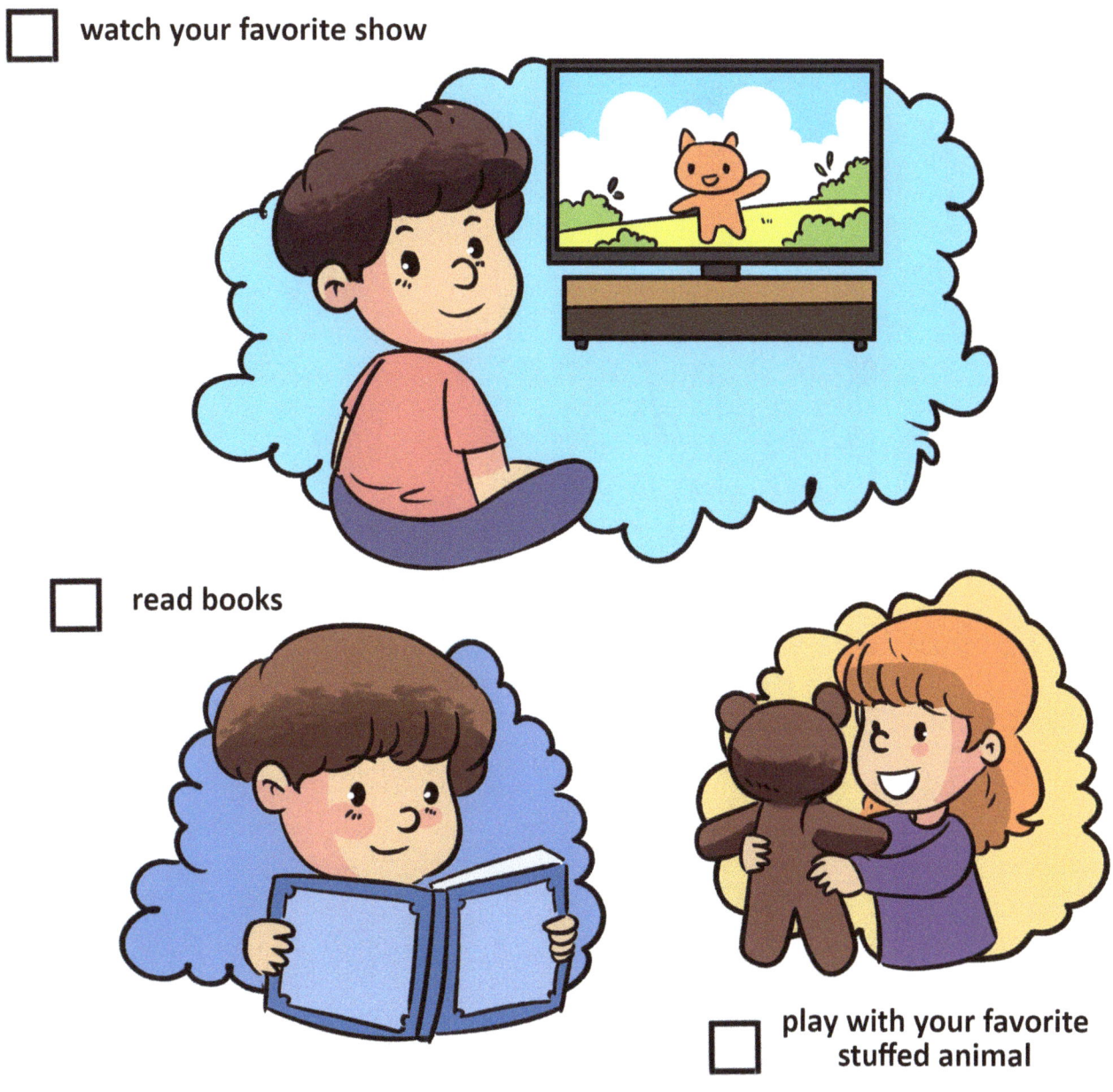

Soon, you will see your doctor to make sure you are healing well and that you're feeling better and getting stronger.

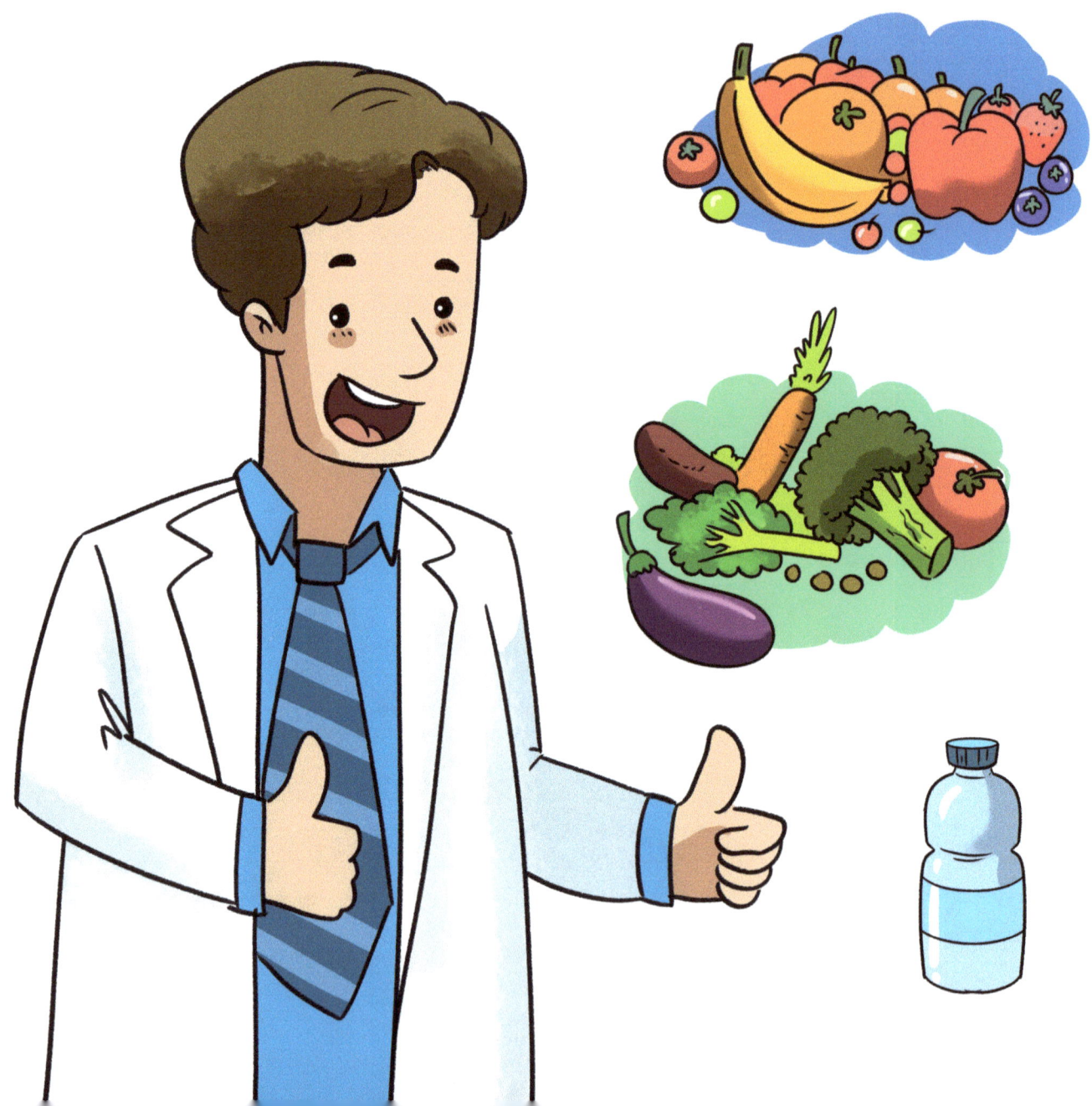

If you have any questions, feel free to ask your doctor.

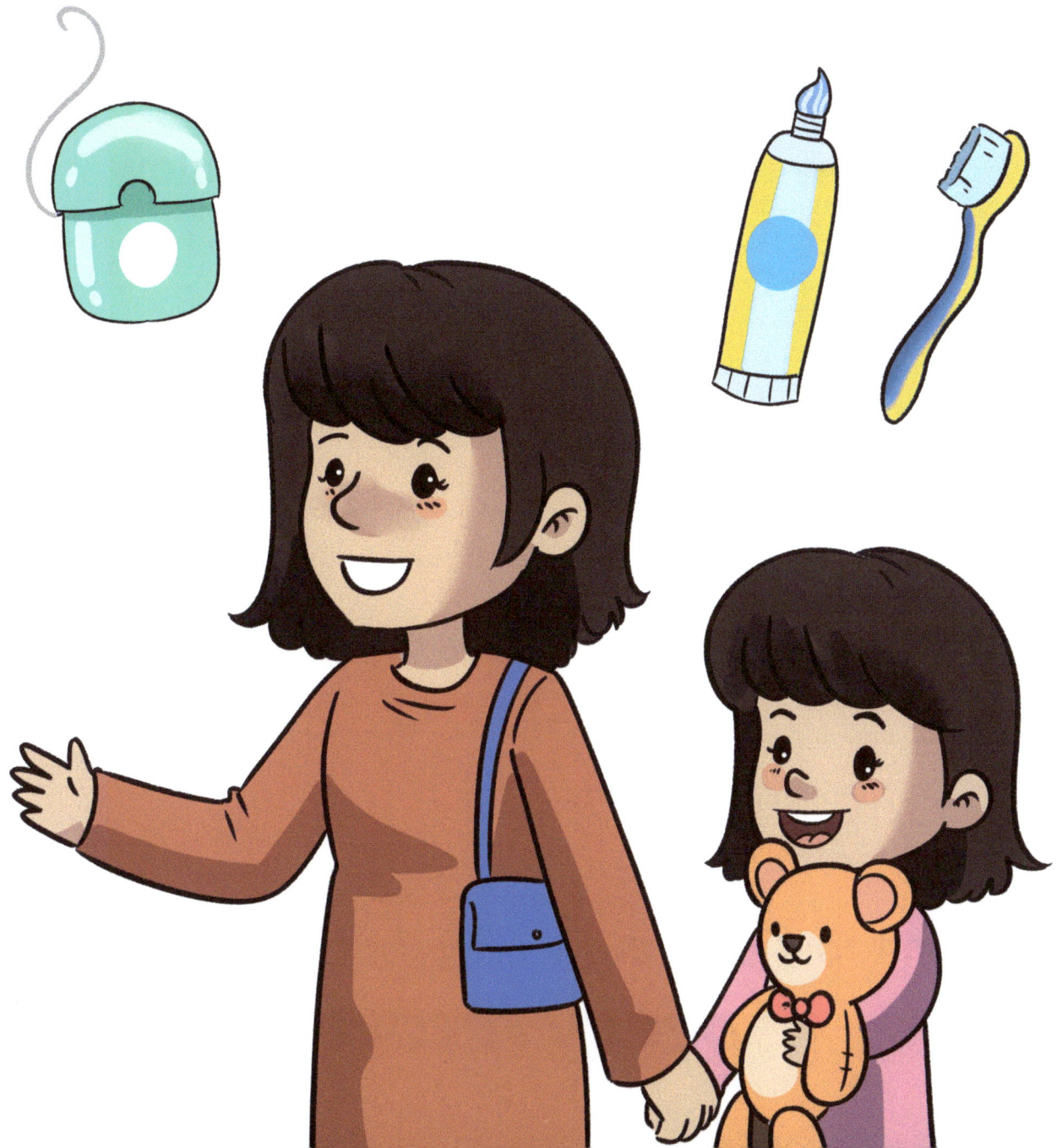

What will you do after your dental surgery?

A party? A celebration?

What's your favorite way to celebrate?

Draw or write your party plan below.

Don't forget to show off your beautiful smile.
Speedy recovery!

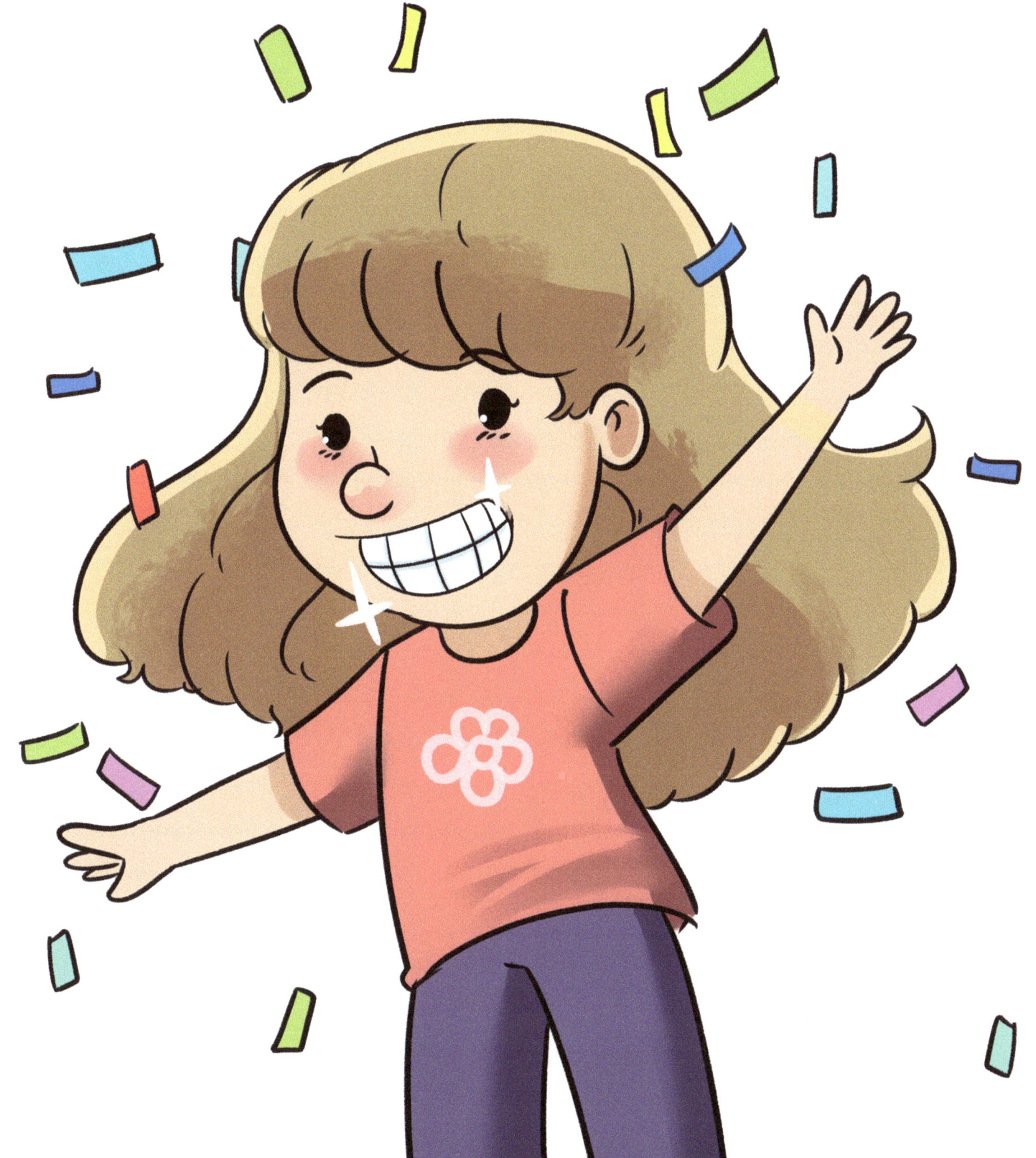

Notes for Parent/Guardian

• Placement of the intravenous (IV) catheter in this young age group is typically done <u>*after*</u> your child is asleep in the operating room.

• Dental surgery may require nasal intubation. This is where a breathing tube is placed through a nostril down to the windpipe, bypassing the mouth and giving the dentist or oral surgeon more space to perform the surgery. No matter how carefully and gently the breathing tube is placed, bleeding in the nose is still likely to occur. In the majority of cases, the nosebleed is mild and limited. It may be helpful to remind your little one that, "It doesn't mean anything is wrong. It's your nose saying, "I'm healing. Please be gentle with me.""

• Post-surgery instructions/restrictions:
Your child's doctor should give you specific instructions on (1) what your child can and cannot do during the recovery period, (2) the duration of the post-surgical restrictions, and (3) any post-surgical follow-ups. Additionally, (4) they should instruct what to watch out for and when it is necessary for you to bring your child back to the hospital in case of an emergency. If they forget, please kindly remind them and obtain these instructions/restrictions before leaving the hospital.

Disclaimer

Please note that the illustrations are not drawn to scale.

This book is written for informational, educational, and personal growth purposes and should not be used as a substitute for medical advice.

Please consult your child's doctor if they need medical attention and to ensure the information in this book pertains to your child's medical condition and needs. I cannot guarantee what your child experiences is exactly what is being discussed in this book.

The author and the publisher are not responsible, either directly or indirectly, for any damages, monetary losses, or reparations due to information in this book. By reading this book, the readers agree not to hold the author and the publisher responsible for any losses as a result of any errors, inaccuracies, or omissions in this book.

Please keep in mind that your child's experience depends on the location, the facility, their medical condition, and the healthcare team. Please use this book in conjunction with your child's doctor's advice. Thank you.

Did this picture book help your child in some way?
If so, I would love to hear about it!

www.amazon.com/gp/product-review/B0FJCST7CL

For other book titles, please visit:

www.fzwbooks.com

Connect with the author

email: books@fzwbooks.com
facebook/instagram: @FZWbooks

Books by the author

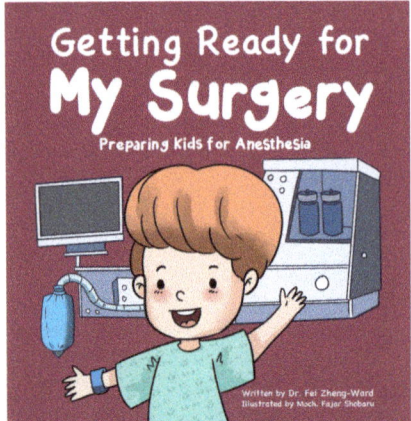
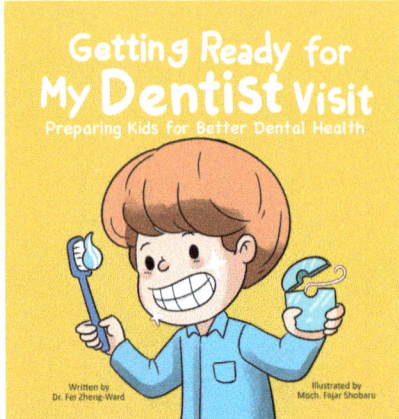
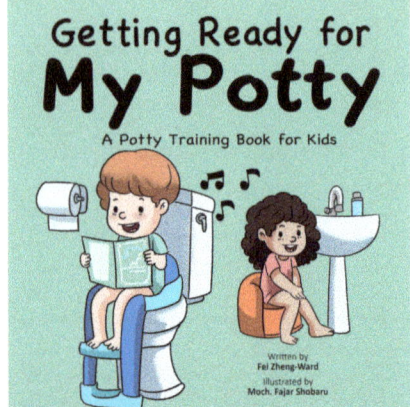
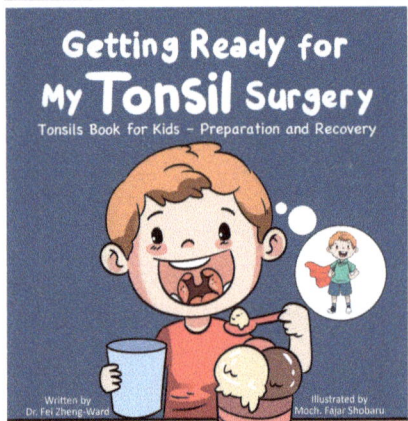
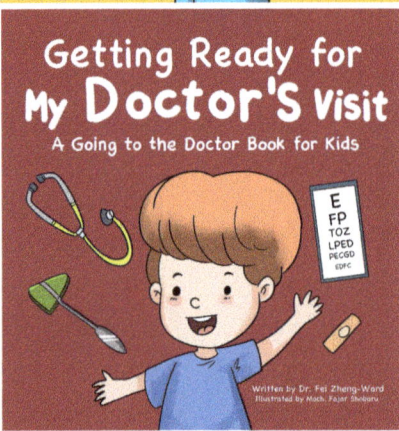
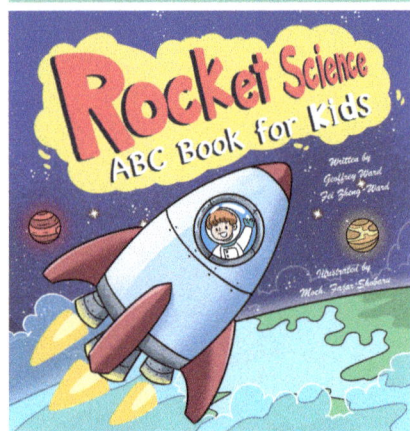
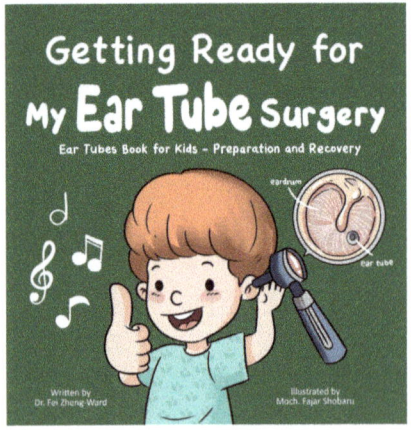
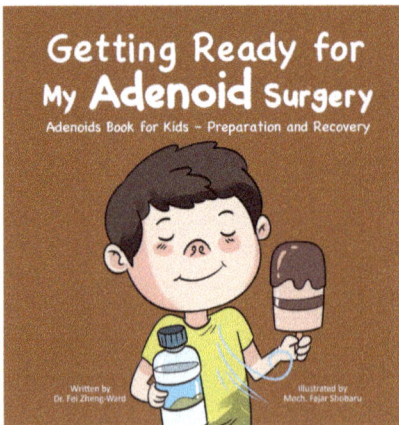
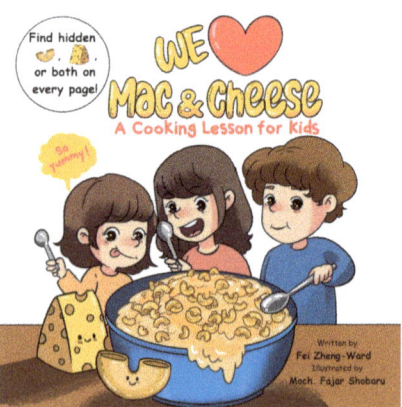

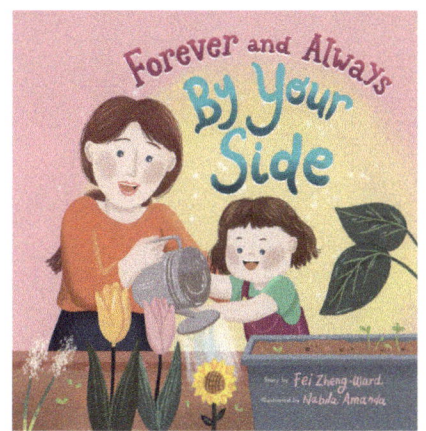
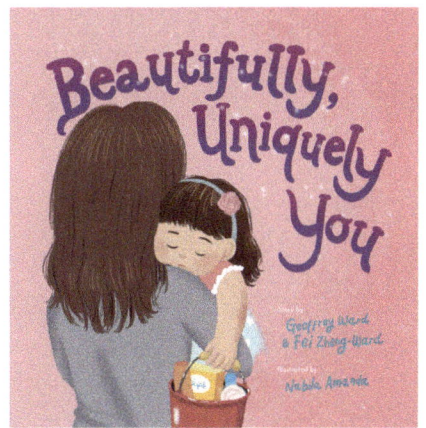
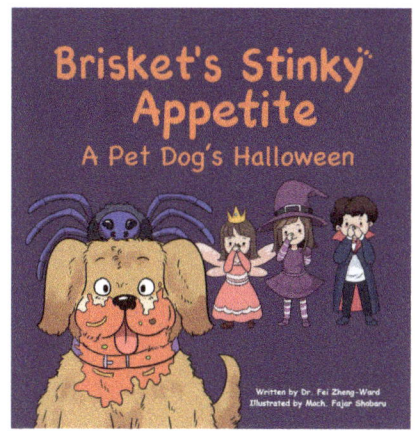
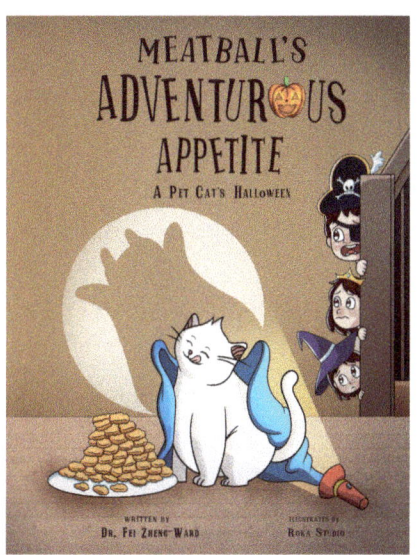
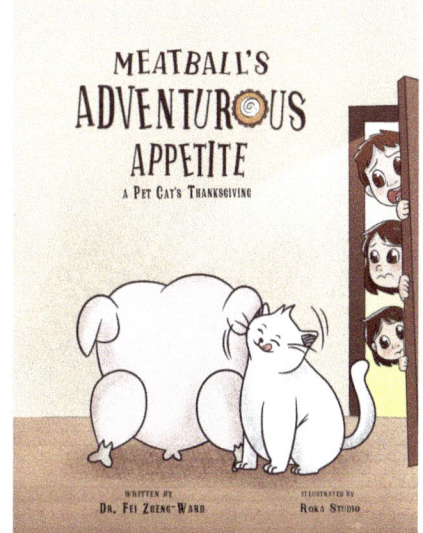
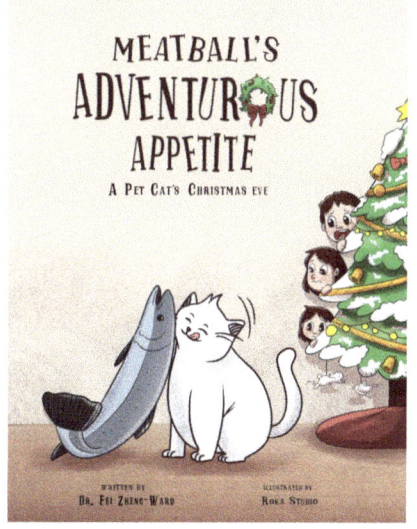
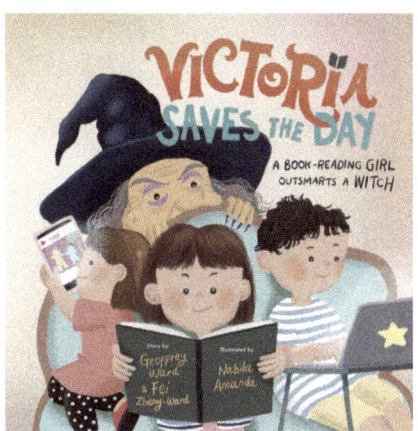
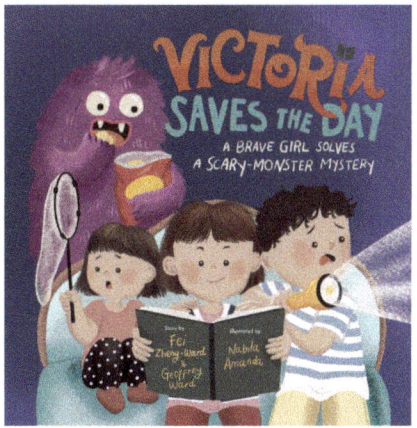
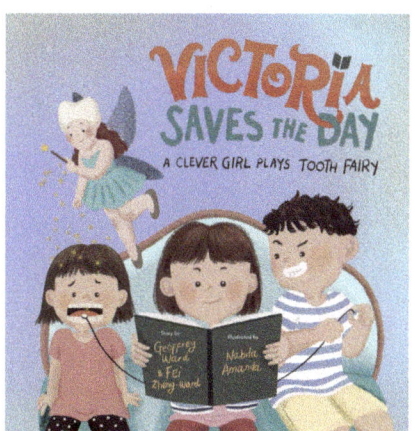

www.ingramcontent.com/pod-product-compliance
Lightning Source LLC
Chambersburg PA
CBHW040000040426
42337CB00032B/5169